PUBLIC HEALTH IN CHINA SERIES
Series Editor Liming Li

HIV/AIDS in China Beyond the Numbers

Editor: Zunyou Wu

Associate Editors: Bernhard Schwartländer

Catherine Sozi

Colin W. Shepard

People's Medical Publishing House

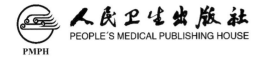

PMPH

Website: http://www.pmph.com/main-en/

Book Title: HIV/AIDS in China: Beyond the Numbers
(Public Health in China Series)
中国公共卫生：艾滋病防治实践（英文版）

Contact address: No. 19, Pan Jia Yuan Nan Li, Chaoyang District, Beijing 100021, P.R. China, phone/fax: 8610 5978 7584, E-mail: pmph@pmph.com

For text and trade sales, as well as review copy enquiries, please contact PMPH at pmphsales@gmail.com

First published: 2016
ISBN: 978-7-117-22864-0

Cataloguing in Publication Data:
A catalogue record for this book is available from the CIP-Database China.

Printed in The People's Republic of China

ISBN 978-7-117-22864-0

9 787117 228640 >

PUBLIC HEALTH IN CHINA SERIES

Series Editor

Liming Li

Chair of Board, Peking Union Medical College/Chinese Academy of Medical Sciences

Professor, Department of Epidemiology, School of Public Health, Peking University Health Science Center

HIV/AIDS in China
Beyond the Numbers

Editor

Zunyou Wu

Director, National Centre for AIDS/STD Control and Prevention

Chinese Centre for Disease Control and Prevention

Beijing, China

Associate Editors

Bernhard Schwartländer

WHO Country Representative China Office

Catherine Sozi

Country Director and Representative UNAIDS China Office

Colin W. Shepard

Country Director, US CDC GAP China Office

People's Medical Publishing House

Contributors

Zunyou Wu, MD, PhD
Director, National Centre for AIDS/STD Control and Prevention
Chinese Centre for Diseases Control and Prevention
Beijing, China

Elizabeth Pisani, MA, MSc, PhD
Visiting Senior Research Fellow
The Policy Institute
King's College London
London, United Kingdom

Anuradha Chaddah, MD, JD, MPH
Beijing, China

Nanci Zhang, MPH
National Centre for AIDS/STD Control and Prevention
Chinese Centre for Disease Control and Prevention

Acknowledgements

The authors are heavily indebted to the interviewees whose voices appear in this book. The value of their experience, expertise and tireless efforts are incalculable in telling the stories of the HIV/AIDS experience in China. They include Longde Wang, Yi Zeng, Xiwen Zheng, Susu Liao, Baogui Zhu, Ruotao Wang, Shaohua Wang, Lin Lu, Xi Chen, Guohui Wu, Xiping Huan, Xinlun Wang, Le Geng, Lingping Cai, Thomas Cai, Lin Meng, Ray Yip, Bernhard Schwartländer and Catherine Sozi. Full interviews with some of these people can be found in *China's Journey fighting AIDS –participant stories*, edited by Wenkang Zhang and published by the People's Medical Publishing House in 2015.

The authors thank Yan Cui, Wei Guo, Dongming Li, Zhengwei Ding, Yurong Mao, Houlin Tang, Ye Ma, Hui Liu and Di Wu for creating figures for the book.

Gratitude goes toYang Hao, Zhenquan Jiao, Wen Jiang, Zhongdan Chen, Na He, Jennifer McGoogan, Cynthia X. Shi, Julio S.G. Montaner and Roger Detels for their comments and assistance for this work, your guidance has been invaluable.

This book would not have been possible without your assistance.

Note: Chinese names are conventionally given with the family name preceding the given names. In this book, we retain that convention for national leaders (for example, President Xi Jinping). Officials, scientists and others are referred to using the Western convention, in which given names precede the family name (for example, epidemiologist Xiwen Zheng).

Acronyms

AIDS	Acquired immune deficiency syndrome
CD4 cell	A type of white blood cell, essential part of the human immune system
China CDC	Chinese Centre for Disease Control and Prevention
CRIMS	Comprehensive Response Information Management System
HIV	Human immunodeficiency virus
NCAIDS	National Centre for AIDS/STD Control and Prevention (China)
NGO	Non-Governmental Organisation
SARS	Severe Acute Respiratory Syndrome
STI	Sexually transmitted infection
UNAIDS	Joint United Nations Programme on HIV and AIDS
US CDC	United States Centers for Disease Control and Prevention
WHO	World Health Organization

Contents

Contents

Contents

Introduction

Zunyou Wu and Elizabeth Pisani

The story of human immunodeficiency virus (HIV) in China over the last three decades has been a gripping one: it is a tale first of exclusion and fear, and then, by turns, of involuntary tragedy, cautious experimentation and finally vigorous response. Above all it has been a story of learning, first by a small group of dedicated doctors and public health specialists who had the courage to face the facts and propose unorthodox solutions, and later on by a broader group of policy makers and social groups. The voices of those most affected by the epidemic have grown stronger over time so that now, thirty years after the first case of acquired immune deficiency syndrome (or AIDS) was identified in China, the country is willing actively to face the challenges of an epidemic that has touched families throughout this vast nation, rather than to deny and marginalize those living with HIV.

This book follows the narrative of China's HIV epidemic in some detail. Reaching beyond the numbers and figures that are often used to outline the impact of HIV on a population, the authors have aimed to take the reader behind the scenes and to bring to the forefront the voices of the scientists and officials on the frontlines of China's experience with HIV. Many of these people have been generous with their time, providing extensive interviews for this book, and you will find them quoted throughout. While their stories and the wider narrative do not always make comfortable reading, everyone involved felt that it was important to give an honest account of these events; they all recognise that the lessons of the past have contributed in important ways to the strength and success of China's response at present.

This book is largely chronologically arranged, with each chapter focusing on a particular phase or aspect of the epidemic or the response. Chapter 1 illustrates how China's social and moral environment at the dawn of the epidemic led its leaders to hope that HIV could simply be kept out of China by excluding foreigners. This hope was shattered with the unexpected discovery of an indigenous HIV epidemic among injection drug users in south-western China. Chapter 2 examines the tragic infection of hundreds of thousands of former plasma sellers in central China. Chapter 3 introduces the AIDS warriors and their early efforts to understand, through carefully designed research, how best to prevent the spread of HIV in the groups at highest risk for infection in China. Chapter 4 examines the factors that catapulted HIV up the political agenda, allowing public health officials and their partners to tackle HIV and risk behaviours more vigorously. The controversial programme of mass testing, which opened the door to more treatment, is the focus of Chapter 5. The next chapter, 6, describes the rapid, nation-wide expansion of both treatment and prevention programmes for those most at risk. The Chinese government moves centre stage in Chapter 7, as it takes strong leadership of a previously fragmented response, while increasing its partnerships with civil society. In Chapter 8, HIV-related stigma, that continues to constrain how the people of China deal with HIV, is discussed. The ninth and final chapter draws together the lessons that China has learned through the ups and downs of its 30-year HIV epidemic.

While the heart of this book takes the reader "beyond" the numbers, the numbers themselves are fascinating and when seen through the eyes of an epidemiologist reveal the ever-changing patterns of HIV infection in China over time and across the nations geographies. An Appendix at the end of this volume provides a detailed account of the 30 years of epidemiological data collected throughout China's epidemic, together with information on funding and service provision. It provides figures and graphs that illustrate the dramatic ways in which the HIV epidemic had changed from its inception to the end of 2015, and shows how expanding services have affected that change.

Though China's experience has been unique in some respects, it is an experience that provides valuable lessons for other countries as they confront their own HIV epidemics. Principal among these lessons is the importance of basing decisions on information that is carefully collected and honestly analysed, rather than on ideology. We hope the examples highlighted in this book will prove useful to those who are curious about the history of HIV in China, as well as to those who are faced with the challenges of preventing the spread of HIV and of caring for those already infected in other parts of the world.

2

Chapter 1

AIDS Comes to China

Elizabeth Pisani and Nanci Zhang

"For infectious diseases, there is no border. Sooner or later we will see AIDS in China."

—Epidemiologist James Chin, Spring 1985, as recalled by Xiwen Zheng

China is a country of superlatives, of "mosts" and "largests", and it's also extraordinarily diverse. Nearly one in every five people on the planet is a citizen of China – an astonishing 1.37 billion people in all. They are scattered across a vast area that spans over 5,000 kilometres and borders on 14 other countries – that gives China more neighbours than any other nation. The people of China are scattered across deserts, lush river valleys, and mountains both tropical and icy, but well over half are now crowded into the country's rapidly growing cities – places that are bursting with ambition and enterprise. The central government and all the most important bodies of the Communist Party that has ruled the country since 1949 sit in the capital Beijing, in north-eastern China. Increasingly, though, the nation's 23 provinces, 4 municipalities, 5 autonomous regions and 2 special administrative regions are taking charge of their own health and welfare programmes. (In this book, for the sake of brevity, we refer to all of these first-level administrative divisions as "provinces".) It is this amazing country that serves as the backdrop to the story that unfolds in the pages ahead.

Few countries in the world have gone through as much social and economic change in the few decades since AIDS first emerged as has China. The changes were already well underway at the start of the epidemic; they had been in motion since the People's Republic of China was founded in 1949. At the time, much of the country was desperately impoverished and its already rudimentary infrastructure was shattered by war. The new socialist government set about rebuilding the country with vigour, and the early focus was as much on social and moral reform as it was on the economy. A great deal was done to promote the equality of women, for example; the last vestiges of polygamy were eliminated and social norms which tolerated men's consumption of commercial sex and predatory relationships with much younger women upended. By the late 1970s, prostitution was believed to be non-existent, and sexually transmitted diseases eradicated, in part thanks to significant efforts to provide healthcare in rural areas through a programme known as "Barefoot Doctors". Susu Liao, an epidemiologist at Peking Union Medical College who once served as a barefoot doctor herself, described the sentiments of the time: "After the founding of the new China, sex workers were deemed downright detestable. The country set about exterminating prostitution and sexually transmitted diseases through campaigns and movements. It was a hallmark of the socialist system that we were rid of the 'obscene'."[1] It goes without saying that there was no place in socialist China for the seemingly depraved behaviours that raged through Western countries in the late 1960s and early 1970s – free love, same-sex relationships and getting high on drugs were all demonised by China's publicizing campaign programs.

When AIDS was first reported in the Unites States in 1981, few in China gave it a second thought. In the minds of the leadership, the behaviours that spread HIV simply didn't exist in the new China. When James Chin, an epidemiologist from the United States, visited China in March of 1985 and spoke about HIV, he asked his audience whether they thought the virus was circulating in the country. "Some didn't know, while others said there couldn't be any AIDS in China because sexually transmitted diseases had already been eradicated," recalled Professor Xiwen Zheng, a prominent epidemiologist who translated for Dr. Chin during a lecture to the Chinese Academy of Preventive Medicine. "Then Dr. Chin replied that infectious diseases did not recognise borders and that 'sooner or later we will see AIDS in China'." While some of the audience were shocked and others were disbelieving, an Argentine American tourist died in Beijing just a few months later, proving the American professor right.

An open window lets in fresh air, and flies

For some, a foreigner dying of a foreign disease was of little consequence. As late as 1987, the official *Beijing Review* magazine said AIDS was unlikely to spread in China because "in socialist China, the main means of spreading the virus – homosexuality, casual sexual contacts and drug addiction – are opposed by both the government and public opinion."[2]

For those who opposed China's increasing openness to the outside world, however, the importation of HIV to China was a nightmare come true. For the first two decades of its existence, the People's Republic of China had been consumed with internal turmoil and remained relatively cut off from the world. That turmoil had, however, carried the country dangerously close to the brink of total economic collapse. When U.S. President Richard Nixon surprised the world by visiting China in 1972, the country's leaders began to recognise that international cooperation might help Chinese citizens climb out of poverty more quickly than the isolationist policies of the past. Slowly at first, and then with quickening speed, China launched itself on the road towards economic reform. The government established special economic zones which welcomed foreign investment in manufacturing, and it began to allow farmers to sell excess produce on the open market. At the same time, the country opened its doors to foreigners. There was an immediate influx of travellers; they came for business as well as for pleasure, and they brought money to pay for both.

This "Open Door" policy was extremely effective in kick-starting the economy, but it also had far-reaching social effects. In the early years of the People's Republic, residency permits tied most Chinese citizens firmly to their village or city of origin. But the new manufacturing hubs, established with foreign capital, needed workers. People began to move, on a massive scale. Migrant workers had cash wages in their pockets, they were released from the social control that comes from living in small communities with people who know one another's business, and they very often congregated in single-sex communities. Male migrants provided a ready market for sexual services. On the other side of the equation, the resurgence of the market economy meant that people needed cash much more than they had done in the early years of the new China, when virtually all basic needs were met by the state. Those who weren't lucky enough to land a job in a new economy driven by foreign investment sought ways to extract cash from their luckier compatriots. Not surprisingly, the long dormant sex trade sprang back to life.

"That's the thing about an open window," observed Zunyou Wu, Director of China's National Centre for AIDS/STD Control & Prevention, paraphrasing the former Chinese leader Deng Xiaoping's famous quote, "It lets in the fresh air, but also the flies and the dust."

One of the "flies" was the HIV virus.

Closing the window

Shortly after a gay foreigner died of AIDS in Beijing in 1985, Chinese virologists identified four HIV infections among haemophilia patients who had received transfusions of blood products imported from the United States. They were tracked down by virologist Yi Zeng, who directed China's sole AIDS research programme at the time. He had witnessed the manufacturers of the blood products showing them off at a medical conference. "Later, they gave the serum to the hosting hospital, Zhejiang Provincial Hospital," he remembered. Local health authorities found that the products had been given to a total of 19 patients between 1983 and 1985. Yi Zeng tested all 19 for HIV and discovered that four were infected. "This was proof that HIV had been brought to China by an infected batch of Factor VIII serum in 1982 and infected the first Chinese citizen in 1983," Yi Zeng said.

The country's first reaction to these early "imported" infections was to slam the door shut to keep out any more flies. Closing their eyes to the social changes taking place around them, the country's leaders reasoned that since Chinese citizens did not themselves engage in the behaviours that spread HIV, the virus could be arrested at the country's borders. Excluding foreigners entirely was no longer an option; at the time, foreign capital and expertise were driving China's economic growth. So authorities sought to exclude the virus itself.

Overnight, China stopped buying blood products from overseas. Irrationally, the import of second-hand clothes was also banned. The next step was to keep out HIV-infected individuals.

"We were asked to draft a working plan to conduct health checks among key population groups while strengthening vigilance at ports in an effort to block AIDS outside the country gate," said Baogui Zhu, who was appointed head of Beijing Institute of Health and Quarantine just a year before the first AIDS case was identified in China.[1] "So we drew up a plan to monitor entry and exit of key population groups at international ports." Anyone found to be HIV-infected was immediately deported. Just in case that plan failed, the government issued regulations forbidding Chinese citizens from having extramarital sex with foreigners.

The first incident Zhu had to deal with involved a foreign hotel manager who tested HIV-positive during a routine medical check. "This was a huge shock to us, since he was not only well known in the industry but also very famous among political circles," said Zhu. "I was told that this manager has very strong connections and I should be cautious when handling this. To which I replied, 'I am the executor of the national law. No matter how much caution I need to exercise, he needs to go'." The multinational company that owned the hotel then sent their regional human resources manager to China for discussions. Zhu recounted what happened next. The first question they posed was, "How reliable is your testing method?" I replied: "We follow the testing method used in the Institut Pasteur labs in France, brought back by Dr. Yi Zeng, our virologist. It is more than reliable." The next round of questions was even more aggressive: "Did you take the blood sample yourselves? Was there any mix-up when drawing the samples? Is it possible that someone else blood was dropped on his head?" Assured that the procedures were completely standardised and that there was no possibility of an error, the company nonetheless insisted on conducting another HIV test itself. Only after that proved to be positive did the hotel manager leave China.

Though these measures may sound draconian these days, it's worth remembering that China was by no means the only country to try to keep HIV-infected foreigners out of its territory. The United States was one of 58 nations that refused HIV-positive people permission to visit; it did not drop that ban until 2010, the same year that China did.

Officials were reacting to the world as they understood it. Westerners were perceived to be the sole source of AIDS, and they were excluded or prevented from mixing sexually with the local population. Chinese citizens were automatically protected by their strong morality: again in the words of the official *Beijing Review*, "homosexuality and casual sex are illegal and contrary to Chinese morality." As late as March 1988, virologist Yi Zeng reiterated the official line. "It's a foreign threat," he said. "The only way for AIDS to come into China is from foreigners." He was right, of course. The virus first mutated into a form harmful to humans outside of China, so the first infections among Chinese citizens must have been contracted from foreign sources. But the assumption that HIV could not spread within China proved to be very wrong. While all eyes were focused on foreigners arriving in big cities, HIV was creeping in through China's back door. It was discovered almost by accident.

Domestic invasion: HIV spreads in Yunnan

The Open Door policy made it easier for people to trade back and forth across China's land borders. This was a relief for the indigenous groups of south-west China and the northern Mekong region. Historically, the residential and working spheres of these groups had spanned the border areas; however, the strong border control imposed during the early years of the People's Republic of China had severely restricted their movements. Such restrictions were inconvenient, but they had one effect that many saw as positive: they insulated Guangxi, Sichuan and Yunnan provinces from most of the worst by-products of the war waged by the United States against the North Vietnamese in the 1960s and 1970s. One of those by-products was heroin. With the relaxation of border controls, the drug began to find its way into China.

Opium poppies had long been grown in the region, and many indigenous people in rural areas smoked and ate opium. But as refined heroin, initially manufactured largely for consumption by US troops during the Vietnam War, began to trickle in across the Burmese border into China's south-westernmost province of Yunnan, people started to inject it. The public security bureau (China's police force) knew about this. They responded by monitoring drug users and setting up compulsory detoxification centres. Police data suggested that by the end of the 1980s, up to 3% of the population in border areas were addicted to opiates, and an increasing proportion of them were injecting.

In 1989, Ying Ma, an epidemiologist who worked for Yunnan Centre for Disease Control and Prevention and specialised in hepatitis control, began to worry about the role that this switch to injecting might play in spreading Hepatitis C. Since she had good relations with the local police force, she asked for permission to draw blood from drug users in detoxification centres for a survey of hepatitis. On testing the samples, she was shocked to find that 95% of them tested positive for Hepatitis C. Almost as an afterthought, she decided to test the blood for HIV as well, even though, except for the four haemophilia patients described above and one person returning from Hong Kong, the virus had never been found in a Chinese citizen.

Two out of every five samples tested positive for HIV.

It seemed absolutely impossible that 40% of drug users in one of the remotest areas of China could have been infected with this "foreign" virus. There must be some mistake, thought Ying Ma. She went back, took another set of blood samples, and found similar results. Immediately, she alerted Beijing, asking for help from the few HIV experts that then existed in China.

The epidemiologist Xiwen Zheng and two of his colleagues responded as swiftly as they could, flying to the provincial capital Yunnan and then travelling to the remote border area of Ruili by bus. The five-day bus journey through the sparsely inhabited mountains of south-west China increased their scepticism about the reported HIV outbreak. The unvarying narrative in China had been that HIV was a virus that came with nightclubs and gay bars and the loose morals of modern urban life. It just didn't seem possible that AIDS could exist in these sparsely populated green hills, with their rutted roads and bamboo-hut villages. But when they reached Ruili and repeated the testing, the researchers found 146 people living with HIV.

Ying Ma had been right. HIV was spreading among Chinese citizens, not in big cities but in the remotest,poorest rural villages. This required a radical rethink, according to Ruotao Wang, who participated in the earliest investigations of the Yunnan epidemic on behalf of the Chinese Centre for Diseases Control and Prevention (China CDC). "AIDS, a disease previously thought to happen only in capitalist countries, was now spread to our farmers in our own land. The people first infected with HIV in Ruili, Yunnan, were all everyday people. They were not foreign travellers. They were all ordinary people who got infected. There was nothing capitalist in the spreading of this epidemic."

No one knew quite how to react to the news. The first instinct of the local government was simply to deny what was happening. The discovery of this highly stigmatised disease was terribly embarrassing for local authorities, an indication that they had not been able to uphold the moral standards of the new China. The epidemiologists and virologists had to visit and plead with them three times before they agreed that the information could be passed on to national authorities. Zheng, who was responsible for providing expert advice on the epidemiology of HIV to the government, recalls being invited to the State Council's headquarters in Zhongnanhai, next to the Forbidden City in Beijing, to report on the outbreak. "At the time the number of HIV-positive people in Ruili had reached 146. There had been a total of only 22 cases in the whole country up to that point, so there was a lot of concern about what number to make public. Later I heard that some leaders suggested going for 15 in the public announcement." This under-reporting was by no means unprecedented. Zheng immediately remembered an earlier case in which the real number of cases in an infectious disease outbreak was divided by 10 for public consumption. "The leaders must have meant well, mindful that the people might get scared," he said. "Of course the Ministry of Health and other experts insisted that this was not a good idea and that it was best not to set a fake precedent." In the end, the experts and the politicians came to a compromise. They agreed to announce the real number, but not until after Chinese New Year, so that the people may have a carefree New Year's celebration. Recounting the episode two and a half decades later, the epidemiologist was almost amused: "When I think about how the current number is 810,000 and prevention and control work is going just fine, all that fuss back then seemed a little ridiculous," he said. "However it was the reality, and the leaders were not to blame. It was just that so little was known about AIDS."

Beijing immediately instructed local health officials to set up HIV surveillance among drug users in all regions where the behaviour was known to exist. Early testing in neighbouring provinces, including Sichuan and Guangxi, found no HIV infections, but authorities remained on the alert.

The next step was to try and understand more about what was really happening – exactly how was HIV being transmitted in Yunnan, and how could it best be prevented? Virtually nothing was known about the social or behavioural landscape in which the virus was spreading. Since very few officials in Yunnan wanted to think about the HIV epidemic at all, social scientists based in Beijing teamed up with international organisations to try to understand what was really going on.

In 1991, a small team of investigators visited Nong Dao, a township on the border with Myanmar, close to the area where the first HIV outbreak had been identified. What they found shocked them profoundly. Coming from Beijing and steeped in the narrative of socialist progress, these researchers believed that drug addiction was among the "social evils" that had been eradicated in the new China. "It had been reported that drug abuse reappeared in Yunnan in late 1980s after a long halt, which triggered the HIV epidemic," said Ruotao Wang. "Our research found that this was inaccurate. Drug abuse had never ceased in the Yunnan border areas. In the years after liberation, a few people used to grow opium in their own backyard and used it as a medicine. Local people described opium as an excellent medicine for diarrhoea and aches." What did change was the form in which people took the drugs. In the late 1980s, refined opium in the form of heroin (known locally as "White Powder" or "Number 4") appeared on the local market. "White powder was expensive," explained RuotaoWang, "so people started to inject it. Now some of the residents along Sino-Myanmar border were very closely mixed, with young men and women often meeting at the market. When taking the white powder they often shared one syringe. It became cool to share a syringe, to show that they were pals."

This syringe sharing, of course, was a very effective way of spreading HIV.

The researchers also noted the local government's response to the new wave of drug use. "With extremely limited resources, the local government nevertheless fought their 'war against drugs' with tenacity," said epidemiologist Susu Liao, another member of the investigation team. "I can still picture the rehabilitation centre in Nong Dao: in a big courtyard, there were these very simple brick stoves; every single addict forced to get clean here had to cook for himself using the rice brought by his family. In other words, rehabilitation here was not just a painful 'hard quit', it couldn't even provide for basic subsistence of the admitted patients." The psychological environment also left something to be desired.

Compulsory detoxification centres have been established in China, intended to decrease drug use, and thus, the spread of HIV. However, the effectiveness of these centres has not yet been fully examined through research studies. A stint in detoxification rarely results in a former addict giving up drugs. "Having lived under this forced rehabilitation, many addicts went out looking for drugs the first thing after leaving rehabilitation," reported Ruotao Wang. In later research, the staff of one rehabilitation centre reported that one addict had come back to the centre 35 times. Eight out of ten relapsed at least once, and over half were back in involuntary detoxification within a year.[3] Getting together with friends to inject after release from a term in detox, drug users – most of whom were male – would be very likely to pass on any newly acquired infection. And since HIV is transmitted sexually most easily soon after a person is first infected, a reunion with a wife or girlfriend or a spree in a brothel after release also carried the risk of passing the virus on to people who were not themselves drug users.

These early studies in Yunnan shattered the myth that HIV could not spread in China. They also clearly demonstrated that the current approach to addiction rehabilitation was not working. Researchers woke up very quickly to the fact that in terms of reducing addiction as well as preventing the rapid spread of HIV, a new approach was needed. Chapter 3 describes the steps they took to try and help China's leaders wake up to those same harsh facts. The process was slow and meticulous. And it was interrupted in the mid-1990s by a catastrophe that made the shock of the Yunnan drug-injector epidemic look almost insignificant, that forced the HIV epidemic in China into the international limelight and that eventually led to the country's comprehensive response. That catastrophe, described in the next chapter, was the mass transmission of HIV among farmers who made money by selling their blood.

Chapter 2

Selling Blood Spreads HIV

Anuradha Chaddah and Zunyou Wu

"Selling plasma to blood product companies infects a large number of donors on one single occasion, if only one is infected"

—From "HIV/AIDS: China's Titanic Peril"[4]

The central farmland of early 1990s China saw the average farmer working long hours, rising before dawn and often not returning home until after sunset. Fields were ploughed, planted and irrigated by hand. Compensation for these long days of labour was minimal: the average rural farming household earned between US$8 and US$12 a month, a meagre living eked out from an average of 0.05 hectares of land per person, about the size of two tennis courts. Faced with pressures to feed and educate one's family, and to ensure the successful marriage of one's children (often an expensive proposition), the farm labourer was in a position of particular financial vulnerability. It was through this fragile population that the commercial plasma donation industry ploughed a disease-ridden trench leading to the infection of thousands with HIV.

Plasma collection in China

The demand for human blood and its components as a critical part of modern medical care has always been high. Whole blood is used primarily for clinical transfusion in people who have suffered blood loss. Plasma is the pale yellow liquid component of whole blood, in which various proteins, electrolytes, lipids, amino acids and vitamins are dissolved. Plasma provides the raw materials for more specialised blood products such as albumin, intravenous immunoglobulin and blood-clotting factors. In general, the human blood market has been divided along procurement and compensation lines between the whole-blood market and the plasma market. In most countries whole blood collection, in which blood is extracted from a donor and used in its totality, is largely collected on a voluntary basis with no financial remuneration for the donor. On the other hand, blood plasma is a highly lucrative commercial product that is collected from paid donors, providing significant financial reward for donors, pharmaceutical companies and the middlemen plasma collection agencies that forge the relationship between these two parties. Blood plasma is procured by first collecting whole blood from a donor, taking that whole blood and separating the plasma component from the cell component via centrifugation. This is followed by the extraction of the freshly separated plasma component, with the remaining red blood cell component then returned intravenously to the donor.

The process of plasma collection was first used in the early 1950s to treat an American patient with autoimmune disease. By the 1970s, the practice had become widely accepted around the world; it was first introduced into China in 1979. At that time, the country already had a 30-year-old paid whole-blood donation system. The government tried at this juncture to end the paid blood collection system in favour of voluntary donation; however, this met with little success as the public did not readily accept the idea of simply giving away this newly valuable commodity. Cultural factors also played a role in dampening enthusiasm for voluntary blood donation. Traditionally, loss of blood is not only seen as being extremely detrimental to one's health but, worse yet, is considered an act of disloyalty to one's ancestors whose blood one has carried into this life.

While blood donations decreased in China, the demand for related medical blood products did not. Not only was there not enough blood being collected domestically, supply of these blood products was also compromised by the fact that there were very few blood product pharmaceutical companies that had the technology to transform raw materials (donated blood) into the clinically valuable end products (immunoglobulins, albumin etc.) needed by the country. China was therefore heavily dependent on imported clinical blood products. This would soon change with the emergence of HIV/AIDS onto the global scene in the early 1980s.

The rise of plasma selling

As was noted in the previous chapter, China's initial reaction to the earliest reports of HIV/AIDS and the unfolding epidemic in the U.S. was to characterise it as a disease of foreigners. The first known case, discovered in a foreign tourist, was quickly followed by the diagnosis of HIV in Chinese haemophilia patients who had been transfused with foreign blood products, specifically factor VIII. These cases were seen as a signal that foreign blood products were inevitable vectors for HIV and subsequent AIDS. In a move to prevent HIV from entering China, the Chinese government banned the import of all foreign blood products. This strategy, aimed at securing the safety of the blood supply, created a dramatic shortage of medically needed blood products. This shortage, and the subsequent response, gave rise to the full-blown commercial plasma selling, a system that would prove to be responsible in large part for China's future HIV crisis.

China's commercial plasma selling emerged in the early 1980s. Equipped with newly imported blood collection machinery and technology, plasma centres began opening across the country. They were particularly concentrated in poorer, rural communities, largely in central China, where paid plasma donation was seen as a viable income source for low-wage farmers. In Henan province, for example, a central province south of Beijing with a population at the time of 70 million and a significant agricultural base, some 200 registered plasma collection centres were opened in less than one year. This is an incredibly large number of collection centres for an area of this size. By comparison, today China has less than 500 collection centres across the entire country.[5,6] Henan's centres were used extensively; in one village a reported 42.8% of adults below the age of 60 participated in blood donation, while another village with a population of fewer than 2,400 residents had, at the peak of the plasma selling, up to six blood-collection stations in service.[7] Local governments approved as many blood collection centres as possible; the necessary systems for monitoring centre operations, however, were rarely put in place.

Pharmaceutical companies were delighted by these developments. China's rural communities were regarded as largely free of drugs and prostitution, and thus good sources of "clean" plasma. Despite the existence of strict regulations governing the amount of plasma that could be donated by any given individual and the frequency with which those donations could occur, very few local health authorities had the actual means to enforce them. Without meaningful oversight or a system of accountability in place, plasma centres were free to focus on profits, sometimes disregarding donor safety or the safety of the plasma supply itself.

Most paid plasma donors were adults between the ages of 20 and 50. They were paid the equivalent of US $6 per 400 millilitres of plasma donation, a considerable sum relative to the average monthly farming income of between US $9 and US $12. Driven by a desire to earn higher incomes, donors willingly risked their health by donating more frequently than was allowed under government regulations. The required waiting period between plasma donations was at least 15 days, but many donors sold their plasma twice a week, and some reported that they had blood taken as frequently as every other day.[8] The plasma donation centres themselves, eager to generate even larger revenues, often turned a blind eye to these too-frequent donors and to the common donor practices of using false names and visiting multiple collection centres in order to avoid the mandated minimum 15-day interval between donations.

Further jeopardising the health status of these plasma donors was the lack of adequate infection prevention and control. Blood was often collected under non-sterile conditions within the plasma collection centres themselves, as well as outside of the plasma collection centres where illegal collections occurred in donor's homes and even in their fields. Additionally, donors were often not screened for infectious diseases such as viral Hepatitis B and C, although this was required by the government regulations, and they were certainly not screened for HIV since this was not mandatory until after 1995. During blood collection, blood from up to ten donors of the same blood type was combined into one communal collection bag. This mixture was then centrifuged to separate the plasma from the remainder of the blood.

The plasma, in turn, was poured into a "public plasma" bag that was forwarded to the pharmaceutical companies. The remaining red blood cells, pooled from up to ten different donors, was re-injected into the donors intravenously in order to ward off impending anaemia. With one cycle of plasma donation, a single donor was exposed to the unscreened blood of no fewer than nine other individuals – and likely exponentially more, given that tubing and machinery used in the process were often contaminated from previous donation cycles. This combination of non-sterile collection conditions and non-screened plasma donors would prove to be lethal.

Early cases of HIV in plasma sellers

In the autumn of 1994, a Shanghai-based blood product company performed a random quality assurance survey of their products and received a report that plasma collected from a 41-year-old female donor (Mrs. L) from Fuyang prefecture in Anhui province had tested HIV-1 antibody positive. The company passed this information, along with the donor's name, to the relevant blood collection centre in Anhui, but staff at the local collection centre failed to understand the significance of the "HIV-positive" finding and ignored the report. Two months later, the Shanghai-based blood products company once more contacted the Anhui blood collection centre to inform them again that Mrs. L's blood plasma had repeatedly tested HIV-positive.

Mrs. L's case was the first ever identified case of an HIV-positive individual in all of Fuyang prefecture, an isolated place with few visitors and little commercial traffic. The residents of this rural area were poor farmers with little exposure to the world beyond their villages, and almost certainly without exposure to news or information regarding HIV. Local health authorities immediately sought to understand how this mother of three children had contracted the disease. Investigators in February and March of 1995 screened Mrs. L, her husband, her son and two teenage daughters and discovered that the two men were HIV-negative, whereas all three women were HIV-positive. The women all denied having any history of intravenous drug use, of having received blood transfusions or of having undergone any medical or dental surgeries. Upon learning that all three females in the household were HIV-positive, local authorities immediately assumed that the women were commercial sex workers. However, Mrs. L denied engaging in extramarital sexual relations and her two daughters denied any history of sexual intercourse, a claim later confirmed by comprehensive physical examination.

Little was understood about HIV; not only were the villagers ignorant as to the existence of this disease, the local health authorities themselves knew very little about how HIV was spread outside of the sexual transmission route. These local health officials had no access to international medical literature, and they did not suspect that the blood donation system was a possible culprit in the spread of HIV. An important but troubling breakthrough occurred only after the Anhui CDC called in a former employee who had gone to the United States to complete a PhD in HIV epidemiology at the University of California at Los Angeles (UCLA). That researcher was Zunyou Wu, now Director of the National Centre for AIDS/STD Control & Prevention (NCAIDS) at China CDC; he was in his native town in Anhui writing up his PhD thesis when the call came. Drawing on his knowledge of the recorded association between paid blood collection programmes and infectious disease epidemics in other parts of the world, he found out that the three women had frequently sold plasma, while the two men had never done so.

A site inspection of the local blood collection centre revealed numerous opportunities for contamination during the plasma collection process. Equipment, including scissors, was not sterilized between donations, contaminated cells were re-infused into several donors, and the centre's staff had not received any training in sterilisation techniques. Shockingly, when the centres plasma stores underwent HIV antibody testing, greater than 40% of the collected plasma samples were HIV-positive.[9] The investigative team concluded that Mrs. L and her daughters had become infected during their time as commercial plasma donors, most likely due to contaminated plasma collection equipment and procedures; they could only speculate as to how many other commercial plasma donors across the country were facing the same fate.

Early warning signs of the epidemic to come: seen but not heeded

Almost simultaneously, other HIV-positive plasma donors were identified in the neighbouring province of Hebei. In December 1994, a 47-year-old from rural Yongqing County who had been selling plasma for seven years screened positive for HIV at the Tianjin Blood Bank. When the positive test was confirmed three months later, the Tianjin Anti-Epidemic Station carried out a quick serological survey of 50 plasma donors from the same area. Fully 37 of them were HIV-positive.[1]

At the same time, HIV infections were being diagnosed among commercial plasma donors in Hebei's southern neighbour, Henan. In all three provinces, local health authorities in the areas with identified HIV-positive donors moved swiftly to shut down all plasma collection centres within their local jurisdictions, understanding that each additional day of delay could result in potentially thousands more being infected with HIV. In March 1995, nationwide action was taken when the Ministry of Health ordered all blood product collection and supply centres to cease their operations immediately. Illegal plasma donation centres continued to operate, however, and that a black market in blood products continued to pose a significant public health threat.

While the rapid shutting down of the commercial plasma industry certainly helped curb the numbers of newly HIV-infected plasma sellers, this was only one step that authorities at the time would have needed to take to shut down the HIV epidemic among people who sold plasma. All future plasma sellers would need to be tested for HIV, and collection centres would need to be properly licensed and much more rigorously controlled and inspected to ensure the safety of future blood collection efforts and future donors. Preoccupied with taking the necessary action, the government failed comprehensively to address the health needs of existing plasma sellers, many of whom were now infected with HIV. There was no active HIV testing among people who had sold plasma, and health officials had no idea how many of them were infected and in potential need of services. But they ought to have known that the number was large. Based on the sheer number of unscreened people who sold plasma as well as the number of under-regulated plasma collection centres that were operating during the peak of the plasma selling, no one could have thought Mrs. L, her daughters and the other early cases of plasma-donation-related HIV were isolated cases. They were clearly markers of an already existing HIV outbreak within the commercial plasma donor population.

A few early, small-scale studies undertaken by local health authorities in rural Anhui suggested that the HIV-positive rate in former plasma sellers ranged between 9.1% and 12.5% and found that the likelihood of being infected was positively correlated to the frequency of plasma donation.[8] While many local health officials in paid-plasma donor catchment areas worked to understand the extent of the epidemic, a few were less active, fearing that an HIV epidemic would jeopardise not only business prospects but also their own jobs.

The nascent epidemic remained largely unknown to the vast majority of the Chinese public and to central authorities.

By not trying to identify all former plasma sellers with HIV in the mid-1990s, the health authorities left unknown numbers of HIV-positive plasma donors unaware of their HIV status. These individuals thus went without the counselling and education necessary to prevent spreading of the disease to their sexual partners and unborn offspring. Local, limited disease surveillance already was demonstrating the potential lethality of disease-unaware HIV-positive plasma donors. One epidemiological survey found that in a population of former plasma sellers with an HIV-positive rate of 12.5%, the rate of HIV among their non-donating spouses was 2.1%. In this same population, a localised education campaign promoting the use of condoms was shown to limit the sexual transmission of HIV among the spouses of plasma donors.[10]

Scientists involved in those local surveys were deeply concerned by the rates of infection that they were uncovering. The epidemiologist Xiwen Zheng, who conducted early investigations in Shanxi and Henan, both provinces where paid blood donation was common, found rates of infection that he describes as "gravely high".

Despite the best efforts of these scientists, no immediate efforts were made at a national-level to increase HIV/AIDS awareness in former plasma sellers, to promote voluntary testing of that population, or to provide medical and social support to those infected and to their families. By the early part of the new millennium, the danger of missing this opportunity became painfully evident as thousands of rural villagers began to develop advanced cases of HIV/AIDS.

The emergence of AIDS Villages: the media as catalyst for HIV/AIDS policy changes in China

In late 1999, Jicheng Zhang, a reporter with the *Henan Science and Technology Daily*, found himself on a train headed to the provincial capital. During this train ride, he met two local farmers and their wives who were headed to Beijing to seek treatment for a "strange illness" that was overtaking their home village. The passengers told Zhang of an illness that had no name or evident cure and that had disabled many in their hometown. Desperate for relief, the community had pooled its funds and paid for four of their neighbours to make the journey to Beijing in order to seek expert medical assistance. These villagers were from Wenlou, Henan province.

Eager to investigate this troubling story, Zhang decided to travel to Wenlou to verify the accuracy of the story and to better understand the situation. He was concerned that the villagers' strange disease might be HIV/AIDS, a disease that up until that point had been associated solely with foreigners, drug addicts and prostitutes. He thus took the precaution of being injected with an antiviral medication before embarking on his trip to rural Henan. This was medically entirely useless, of course, but it was good a measure of the poor information available even to the country's intellectual elite. Once in Wenlou, Zhang discovered the truth: the village was overrun with the sick and the dying. When questioned by Zhang, local health officials denied that there was any problem in Wenlou and brushed aside reports by the locals that Wenlou's neighbouring villages were just as badly affected. Zhang reported this in an article published in January of 2000 in the *Huaxi Dushibao*, a newspaper printed in western Sichuan province for fear of reprisals by local officials. His story was picked up by local media outlets and reprinted regionally, but was not picked up nationally by the Xinhua News Agency or the *China Daily*. Zhang's report was the first published media account of HIV/AIDS in rural China and proved to be the start of the media's role in bringing the issue to the attention of the Chinese public, the central government and the global community.

The Chinese media persisted in covering the rural HIV epidemic and its origins in the plasma selling. In February of 2000, the first scientific study specifically linking the spread of HIV/AIDS to plasma donation was published in the *Chinese Journal of Epidemiology*.[11] This study suggested that up to 25% of all former commercial plasma donors could be HIV-positive. *The Southern Metropolis Daily* reported on 31 March 2000 that police in Shanxi province had arrested eighteen people for donating plasma at a black market plasma collection centre and had seized two tons of blood products. Testing of the arrested individuals revealed that 11 of the 18 were HIV-positive, 16 had viral hepatitis, and 7 had syphilis.[12]

Eventually even the *Dahe Daily*, whose piece "AIDS in Henan" had took the bold step of publishing the entire 25,000-character article in March of 2000. The article vividly drew attention to the desperate plight of the AIDS villages and their inhabitants:

> *...Entering the countryside...we came at last to a world that was strange to us, a world of desperate and lonely people. It was as though we had stepped onto a lonely and uninhabited island. There we faced a child who was about to vanish...*

> *We listened to the helpless cry of this unfortunate child, who like others in his family is shackled with AIDS, and must endure life under fearful and hateful eyes...*

> *In Henan, 200 millilitres of blood infected with HIV changed [this child's] life. It might similarly transform the lives of others...*

> *Most people in Henan still believe HIV-AIDS is a distant concern, but the facts ruthlessly confirm that this demon is among us, in our bustling cities and our quiet countryside...*[13]

Up until this point, all of the reporting on China's plasma donor HIV epidemic had been limited to domestic media whose readership was regional, not national. This changed on 2 August 2000 when the *New York Times* ran the first English language article linking Chinese HIV/AIDS cases to paid plasma donation. In her article "Scientists Warn of Inaction as AIDS Spreads in China", medical doctor and journalist Elisabeth Rosenthal described China's blood plasma black market, the process by which plasma was separated from a donor's whole blood, and how what was "left over" was then mixed with the leftover blood of many other donors and re-infused into the donor. She also cited Chinese experts who expressed concern that China's estimate of the number of HIV-positive persons living within its borders was grossly low. Rosenthal's article focused the attention of the global HIV/AIDS community directly onto China. Following directly on the heels of Rosenthal's article, *China Newsweekly*, a national publication, finally brought China's AIDS epidemic squarely onto the national stage with its 18 August 2000 article titled: "AIDS: The New National Calamity". For the first time, a national publication challenged the Ministry of Health HIV/AIDS numbers and openly criticised the government's response to the epidemic:

> *According to a government report, China had just over 15,000 confirmed cases of HIV-AIDS by 1999. Conservative estimates by experts say that number was probably 500,000...*
>
> *There is still time for prevention and control. But the most frightening thing is cold denial and inaction. Unfortunately this is exactly what many official and government agencies are doing right now...*[6]

Two months later the *New York Times* followed up with another article by Elisabeth Rosenthal that brought Wenlou, the AIDS village that Jicheng Zhang had first learned about from the HIV-positive former blood sellers who had shared a ride on a train with him, to the attention of an international audience. Immediately, health officials and organisations from across the globe began to call for action from Chinese authorities. Chinese central authorities began actively to investigate the epidemic in commercial plasma donors.

In March 2001, a team of senior officials from the Ministry of Health headed to Henan for a field visit. Epidemiologist Xiwen Zheng, who was on the team, described the visit.

"When we arrived, the Party Secretary of Henan province, Mr Li Keqiang, met us. No one from the [local] Health Authority was present. ...I sat next to Mr. Li Keqiang. He was very modest. He asked us about the Henan epidemic in great detail. I shared with him the facts and told him that infection of the paid blood donors took place mainly five years ago, i.e. in around 1995, that they got infected through illegal underground blood collection, that although measures had been taken to eliminate underground blood trade as soon as it was found out, by that time the number of infected victims had already soared to between 50,000 and 80,000 in the whole province. Later I was told that Mr. Party Secretary had shared with the provincial leadership that he had no idea until now how serious the epidemic was." The response was swift: Henan's health authority immediately called a meeting of all chiefs of health bureaus in the province. "Representatives all came with a grave and nervous face. At the meeting I was asked to speak again. I first affirmed the efforts and achievement Henan province made in AIDS prevention and control. Then I pointed out the magnitude of the current epidemic."

During that meeting, the epidemiologist was given what he described as a "secret weapon"– permission to carry out more HIV screening in villages thought to be affected by the crisis. His team got to work instantly, and in less than four days they had collected blood from 3,254 people, around a fifth of whom were former plasma sellers.

"On day three, Mr. Liu, the deputy head of Henan's Centre for Epidemic Prevention, came in person to see if preparation work was done. Much to his surprise, we were almost finished. What they did not expect was that we started before daybreak and went back in the evenings to make sure no one was left out. Initial results were really shocking: HIV infection rates of paid blood donors in the three counties were 34.2%, 44.4% and 15.0% respectively, compared to 2.4% among non-blood donors. The skeleton jumped out of the closet."

While the late 1990s had seen China's plasma donation HIV epidemic purposely held back from the public eye, the media of the new millennium had brought it squarely into the spotlight. National health officials travelled to Wenlou and publicly acknowledged the HIV/AIDS crisis in the village and that the majority of cases had resulted from poorly performed plasma collection. The Ministry of Health acknowledged that the 15,000 cases reported through the health system represented only a small fraction of the true number of HIV infections, and said it estimated that 600,000 Chinese citizens were living with HIV. The crisis sparked a controversial widespread HIV testing campaign, described in Chapter 5, which eventually led to a much better understanding of the national epidemic.

The enduring legacy: families destroyed, stigma entrenched

HIV-positive former commercial plasma donors were found to be living in severely impoverished rural households. Almost completely dependent on manual labour jobs to support themselves, the majority of these individuals eventually became too ill to continue working. Many of them had been their family's primary breadwinners; once they could no longer work, their families found themselves under great financial strain.

Another unique characteristic of the former commercial plasma donor-HIV/AIDS epidemic in China stems from the fact that China's paid plasma selling operated very intensely over a relatively short period of time before being abruptly halted in the late 1990s. This timing element resulted in the epidemic's victims all becoming infected, progressing to symptomatic AIDS and dying at around the same time in a chronologically concentrated manner. The devastating economic and emotional impact upon a small village from suddenly having a significant number of adults falling ill and dying resulted in heightened fear and stigma surrounding HIV. This stigma in turn thwarted efforts to control and treat the disease, a vicious circle that is described in greater detail in Chapter 8. Furthermore, these villages saw the creation of a new social class: AIDS orphans. Unlike other high-risk groups, the former commercial plasma donors were not seen as blameworthy for their plight; rather, the authorities who had not well controlled the plasma selling to thrive were seen as culpable. The civil unrest and instability that ensued were important factors that drove and helped craft the government's response to the plasma donor epidemic.

Cleaning up the blood supply: comprehensive action

Various regulations and laws were successively passed to "clean-up" the country's blood supply and that of blood-derived products. After initially closing down all blood collection centres in 1995, the government allowed for the resumption of blood centre operation under much stricter operating rules. The *1996 Regulations for Management of Blood and Blood Products* limited the legal collection of plasma to certain geographical regions and required annual monitoring of all centres across the nation. Efforts were also made to investigate and close illegal collection centres.

Most significant of all, the government mandated the transition from a paid, commercial blood harvesting system to a voluntary, non-paid blood donation system. In October of 1998 the Law of Voluntary Blood Donation of the People's Republic of China came into effect.[14] Consisting of twenty-four articles, the law starts clearly with the simple statement that "The State institutes a blood donation system." It encourages all healthy individuals aged 18–55 years old to donate blood voluntarily and specifies that collected blood may not be sold to healthcare institutions or pharmaceutical companies. Local health authorities, organisations such as the Red Cross and even the army are all called upon to help facilitate the safe and sterile collection of blood and to promote blood donation via public campaigns. Furthermore, the law provides that any individual or institution that sells donated blood could be subject to a fine of up to CNY100,000 (approximately US $16,100) and criminal prosecution.

In the same month that China legally mandated the establishment of a voluntary blood donation system and illegalised all commercial blood procurement, several of its ministries jointly issued the *Long and Medium Term Plan on HIV/AIDS Prevention and Control(1998–2010)*. This plan served as a guide for all aspects of the government's future interventions as related to HIV/AIDS. Included in this blueprint were strict regulations requiring the testing of all blood and plasma donors for infectious diseases and for similar post-collection testing of all blood and its derivative products. In June 2001, the Ministry of Health's Communicable Disease

Control Division put forth a bolder and more detailed five-year action plan aimed at reducing and preventing the spread of HIV/AIDS. The five-year plan emphasised once again the need to ensure the safety of blood and blood products and to prevent the transmission of HIV/AIDS by both the collection and transfusion of blood. The ministry called for the strengthening of compliance with all regulations on the part of blood collection and transfusion organisations, and for stricter oversight such organisation via tighter licensing requirements and annual auditing procedures. In the several years that followed the promulgation of these various laws and regulations, dozens of blood collection centres were shut down for failing to meet the new requirements. As recently as in 2011, Guizhou province had 80% of all its plasma collection centres closed by the provincial health department. Not citing the exact violations that led to the closures, a Guizhou health official would say only that the move was made in order to "keep the Guizhou residents in better health".[15] It should be noted that despite the government's efforts to fully modernise the blood collection system and to ensure the public safety by imposing strict rules around infection control and prevention, illegal blood centres were not completely eliminated. Commercial blood collection companies continued to find remote and impoverished areas where they could operate on a black market basis. In March 2005, the Ministry of Health reported on the closure of 147 illegal paid plasma centres in the previous year alone.[16]

Ensuring a safe blood supply for medical transfusion and for the production of blood-derived medical products is essential to the practice of modern-day medicine. Approximately 12.3 million units of blood are collected in China annually; about 20% fewer than in the United States. As of 2010, according to official reports, one hundred percent of China's blood is collected from voluntary, unpaid donations and all collected blood has been screened for transfusion-transmissible infections (TTIs) such as HIV, Hepatitis B, Hepatitis C and syphilis. Furthermore, national regulations mandate that plasma is collected only through the use of automated plasma collection machines, which use continuous-flow devices that automatically separate a patient's plasma from their blood and then return the cell fraction directly to the donor. This separation of plasma and the return of the cellular component to the donor happen within a closed system. The donor is not exposed to any other donor's blood or collection equipment.

The effectiveness of these screening and contamination prevention measures is tremendous and exemplified in the rates of Hepatitis C infection in China's blood donors. For those who donated blood prior to 1998, Hepatitis C infection prevalence was greater than 12%. This number has dropped dramatically to 1.71% among blood donors who began donating blood after 1998, following the implementation of the stricter blood collection rules and regulations.[17]As of June 2012, according to the World Health Organization (WHO), there are still 39 countries that were not able to screen all of their blood donations for one or more of the above noted TTIs. China's blood collection system has evolved rapidly since the mid-1980s and serves, overall, as an example of a well-regulated, voluntary blood donation system that other countries can strive to follow.

Even with all that China has achieved, there are still aspects of the system that can be improved. Upgrading to timelier TTI screening assays must continue to happen. A January 2015 *China Daily* article relayed the story of a five-year-old girl from Fujian province who became infected with HIV via a blood transfusion she received in 2010.[18] Although the blood she received had been screened for TTIs, it was screened using a test which detects antibodies to HIV, rather than the virus itself. Such antibodies do not show up in an infected donor's blood until around three weeks following the date of actual infection. If antibody tests are used during this time they will give a negative result, even though the blood contains HIV. RNA-based HIV tests close this "false-negative" window to 11 days, but they were, until recently, rarely used. Following the case reported in January 2015, RNA tests have been provided to every blood bank in the country. As a result, authorities expect a halving of the number of cases in which people contract HIV because they receive infected blood that was tested in the window period and thus incorrectly believe they are uninfected.

The Chinese government will need to remain vigilant in order to maintain a tightly regulated and purely voluntary, non-commercial blood collection system. Blood is in short supply relative to demand; in order for China's blood supply to meet the current national needs, 1–3% of the country's population needs to donate blood annually. As of 2010, 0.84% of the Chinese population donated blood; this increased to 0.92% in 2011. Increasing the number of unpaid donors in China may prove quite challenging, especially as blood donation has not historically been associated with altruism and the idea of social welfare, but rather has been associated with extreme poverty and desperation. When commercial blood and plasma collection was first banned in China, authorities placed the responsibility for recruiting greater numbers of non-paid blood donors on the shoulders of local governments. These authorities often pressured local employers and universities into helping them reach their donation targets by levying fines and monetary penalties if target numbers were not reached. To avoid these penalties, employers would give their staff incentives and even cash – reportedly paying over US$200 in some cases.[19] Recognising the coercive elements of such a system, the Ministry of Health, starting in 2004, began to phase out the mandatory employer-organised donation system. Today, China's blood centres are responsible for recruiting individual, non-paid blood donors. Social and cultural barriers will need to be overcome in order to establish a strong, community-based concept of voluntary, unpaid donation in China. Only in this way will sufficient blood supply stores be maintained and obtained without coercion, which will reduce the risk of any repeat of the awful events detonated by unregulated plasma donation in the mid-1990s and therefore enable China to avoid recurrences of the commercial plasma donor HIV epidemic.

It was a long time before China's government became aware of the full magnitude of the HIV crisis among plasma sellers, and longer still to provide care for those that needed it. Their awakening, and the provision of treatment and care, are described in detail in Chapters 4–6 of this book. China's villagers, for their part, have certainly woken up to the realities of HIV. The *New York Times* journalist Elizabeth Rosenthal, who was present at both extremes of this terrible journey towards knowledge, describes that awakening:

> *On my first visit to East Lake [an 'AIDS Village'], in 2001, a hospital nurse had asked me what caused AIDS and how it spread. Now [in 2011] grandmothers, farmers, and country doctors have become unlikely experts in the molecular biology of this complicated disease. Like the best New York City physicians, they tick off their latest blood measurements of CD4 cells, the disease-fighting immune cells that are depressed by the AIDS virus. They trade rumours about new drugs being developed in Harvard labs the way they once shared theories about harvests.*[20]

Chapter 3

The AIDS Warriors

Zunyou Wu and Elizabeth Pisani

"If you want to understand, you have to go to the front-line. Otherwise all your knowledge comes from the imagination, and that's no help at all."

—Longde Wang, Former Vice Minister of Health

As the preceding chapters have made clear, the first HIV outbreaks in China did not lead to an immediate, high-profile, nation-wide response. This was in part because of straightforward denial, but there were other reasons behind the failure to act. The most important of these was that when HIV first started to spread in a corner of the nation far from the capital, officials simply did not know what to do.

China was only just emerging from a long period of isolation, poverty and very stringent social control. Most officials had little or no experience of issues such as drug abuse or prostitution, let alone of dealing with the diseases that might spread through these behaviours. Communities, wearied by social upheaval and economic need and accustomed to following instructions from political leaders, were in no position to organise themselves to fill the gap. In this chapter, we step back to look at how Chinese scientists worked methodically over 15 years to figure out what could practically be done in China to slow the spread of HIV. The ghastly outbreak of HIV among commercial plasma donors described in the previous chapter diverted the attention of some of these scientists for a little while, but by and large, they plodded on to produce information that would help government and communities make better decisions.

China was not the only country to be confronted with HIV at a time of social and economic turmoil. Few of those other countries, however, were as well provided

30

with scientists willing to take on the challenge. A handful of Chinese doctors were studying in the United States when the disease that became known as AIDS was first identified. One of them was Longde Wang, who went on to become China's Vice Minister of Health. He remembers that time: "In 1981, I was studying at medical college in New York when some young homosexual men were found to be infected with a rare disease that progressed quickly and had a very high fatality rate. No one knew what the disease was. The hospital I studied in held a seminar about it and I attended, but only the basics were discussed. From then on, however, I started to work on AIDS."

Long before the outbreak of HIV among plasma donors described in Chapter 2, China was building up a group of pioneering AIDS researchers. Besides Longde Wang, they included virologist Yi Zeng, clinician Aixia Wang, policy researcher Xinhua Sun and epidemiologist Xiwen Zheng. From the mid-1980s, they were building up knowledge and working to develop a critical mass of people interested in HIV. "This group helped train a good number of younger generation professionals who went on to become the main force in AIDS prevention and control in China," said epidemiologist Xiwen Zheng. In May 1988, the Chinese Academy of Preventive Medicine founded two AIDS-related centres, one concentrating on virology, the other on epidemiology. This was remarkably forward-thinking, given that fewer than two dozen people had *ever* been diagnosed with HIV in China at that point.

This is not to say that AIDS was a political priority; it was quite the opposite. Understanding AIDS was, rather, the preserve of a small but fiercely dedicated group of doctors, epidemiologists and public health officials who saw an opportunity in the relative invisibility of the epidemic; these men and women were China's early AIDS warriors. Since the HIV epidemic was largely unknown to the public and politicians, these warriors had the room they needed to start to fill the knowledge gap about how best to respond to HIV in China without external interference. With little fanfare, the staff of the two centres worked together to put in place a surveillance system to track the spread of HIV, as well as to design small, experimental studies that might help guide future prevention programmes.

Establishing the facts and trying out innovative responses can't be done for free. And yet without the facts, it is very difficult to convince politicians to put money on the table for action. That's especially true when the facts are unpleasant, when they relate to prostitution, sex between men and drug use – the sort of issues politicians in any country in the world would rather not know about.

China's small band of dedicated HIV specialists solved this dilemma very cleverly. They worked in partnership with overseas organisations to increase their own knowledge, then used that knowledge to convince politicians to come up with additional resources.

China's specialists sought to learn as much as they could from foreign experiences. Countries such as Australia, Thailand, the Netherlands and the UK were further down their epidemic pathways than was China; they had already confronted many of the issues that were now arising in China. Though there were many differences between the countries, Chinese researchers realised that they did not need to re-invent every wheel on the HIV-prevention wagon. Over the first decade of the epidemic, public health officials organised a number of extended study tours to learn about the HIV prevention approaches adopted by other countries. The HIV specialists were astute. They quickly realised that health authorities alone could not effectively tackle HIV. Other government sectors, including public security and women's affairs, who were at first less open to experimental programmes involving commercial sex or drug use, were needed for an effective response. The researchers set about finding likely allies in those sectors, and ensured that they were included in visits to other countries where they could witness for themselves the success of non-punitive HIV prevention approaches.

After learning what other nations' experts were doing to tackle their own HIV epidemics, the next step for China's specialists was to partner with foreign researchers to begin to understand the specific situation in China itself. Using funding from a variety of overseas sources, the teams moved quickly from formative research that simply described the landscape of risk behaviour in China to intervention research that experimented with possible solutions for preventing HIV.

Throughout this process, the research community and public health officials engaged with those politicians most likely to be responsive, working with them to influence others who may be more reluctant to take on the sensitive issues of HIV.

The strategy worked well. Results from the very first wave of field research in Yunnan were presented to local policy makers at an HIV workshop paid for by the World AIDS Foundation. World AIDS Foundation is a charitable body that received one quarter of the patent royalties on HIV test-kits developed by French scientist Luc Montagnier and American Robert Gallo, who co-discovered the virus. The Yunnan workshop was a good investment; it created enough concern among local policy-makers that the provincial government began actively to court other international partners who could support programmes of research and training. By the end of the decade, UNICEF, UNAIDS, WHO, the Asian Development Bank, the UK Department for International Development, Australian Red Cross, Oxfam, the Salvation Army, Médecins Sans Frontières, the Ford Foundation, Save the Children and the Amity Foundation had between them invested more than US$4 million in programmes intended to reduce the spread and impact of HIV in Yunnan province.[21]

Making friends: the importance of local allies

As we saw in Chapter 1, the domestic epidemic in China began in Yunnan, a part of the country that culturally and geographically is about as far from the core of researchers in Beijing as it is possible to be. Their early fact-finding missions led very quickly to a realisation that better information alone would not be enough to prod local authorities into a response, especially given the fundamental changes that would be needed.

Take the compulsory detoxification centres for drug injectors, for example, with their harsh conditions and their threatening wolfhounds. These did almost nothing to cut drug use among addicts, and the authorities knew it. Fortunately, the local government was not wed to punitive measures; they simply had very little experience with heroin addiction and didn't know what else to do. They were, however, willing to learn. With backing from the United Nations Economic and Social Commission for Asia and the Pacific, Yunnan's Institute of Mental Illness Prevention and Treatment piloted a very different drug prevention programme in four Ruili villages. "The programme sought to help people stay away from drugs through humanity and community building," said Susu Liao, who had also visited these centres in 1991, interviewing the project doctors. "Their work gave us hope in preventing drugs from further spread. However, shared injection equipment had already opened Pandora's box and released the evil that was HIV."

Programmes such as these have perhaps been unfairly overlooked. Epidemiologist Xiwen Zheng said he found himself repeatedly calling attention to these very early positive steps from a local government just beginning to understand the crisis it faced. He noted that HIV activists at international conferences "were fond of mentioning human rights, asking how China treated drug users infected with HIV/AIDS and whether there was discrimination". In response, he said: "I shared with them how it was done in Ruili in the early days when some drug users were found with HIV: that they lived in a courtyard with some surrounding field designated to them for growing vegetables, that the government made sure their basic living needs were met, that sometimes TVs were provided, that epidemic prevention staff did educational campaigns, and that the family could visit every week. This way, the patients' basic subsistence was met while infection via intravenous injection was reduced." Most importantly, these examples showed that it was indeed possible to find allies within local governments and communities, and even in local police forces. These alliances became very important as this small band of HIV specialists began to experiment with different ways of tackling the epidemic.

Beneath the red lantern: examining the commercial sex trade

In those early years, Chinese health officials also looked around themselves at the course that HIV seemed to be taking elsewhere in Asia. In nearby countries, and particularly in Thailand, they noticed that an initial spike of infection among drug users was very quickly followed by a dramatic increase in the number of female sex workers who were testing positive for HIV. Logically, that meant that male clients were being exposed to the virus. If they became infected, the men who were buying sex could then in turn pass HIV on to their wives or girlfriends. Among women who sold sex in Bangkok, HIV seemed to be climbing inexorably. When prevalence was first measured in 1989, 3% of sex workers were infected with HIV. By 1993, that number had climbed to 28%; it was to stay at those levels for several years. Not surprisingly, since most sex workers become infected by their clients, HIV had also risen sharply among men with risky sexual behaviour in Thailand. Among military conscripts aged 19–21 in northern Thailand, over 80% of whom had paid women for sex, HIV prevalence was 12.5%.[22,23]

Could the same thing happen in China? Across society as a whole, sexual mores were certainly changing. Lovers and courtesans had feature prominently in classical painting, poetry and literature of Imperial China, at least in descriptions of the wealthy mercantile classes, although "loose" sexual behaviour was always officially frowned upon. China's Communist Party had begun work to eradicate these behaviours even before it came to power in 1949.

So it was that when epidemiologist Susu Liao began researching the sex trade in the early 1990s, she was genuinely shocked by what she found. Most researchers expect to be able to "stand on the shoulders of giants", in other words, to build on the work of others who have asked similar questions before them. Liao found almost no research from the previous few decades. "Back then, even scientists and researchers steered well away from topics involving sex, let alone prostitution," she said. "It wasn't until the country's opening up in the 1980s, and especially the arrival of AIDS, that we had to face these marginalised problems which in the past never would have made it into the realm of research."

Her effort to understand what was going on was at first constrained by the people to whom she had access. "We came into contact with the women taken in by the Public Security Bureaus Centre for Female Re-education," said Liao. "What we saw were all re-educated women and what we heard were all stories told by the police. The main impression we had was one of reform, that the society would reform these women and persuade them away from this line of work so that they could support themselves through some other means of living." The success of these efforts was unclear. "The police would tell us, however, that it was hard for these women to switch to another industry."

Liao recounted a failed attempt to collect information in massage parlours in a town in Yunnan. "They told us that the girls are not working now because foreign diplomats were scheduled to visit Xishuangbanna soon. Apparently a deputy chief of Yunnan province had come early to Xishuangbanna's capital Jinghong to ensure that no inappropriate things were in sight. But during his evening walk, he ran into several troupes of working girls trying to solicit business. This was considered detrimental to securing investment in Yunnan– they must be stopped right away. Therefore a major sweeping of the obscene industry began. Girls were not working anymore. The streets were also wiped clean. In front of several massage parlours near our hotel, the word 'massage' on the glass lighting boxes was smashed, leaving broken glass hanging in the doorway. The wooden signs had the word 'massage' painted in white, adding ugly scars to the already rough looking plates. Perhaps the sweeping of the obscene came too urgently to care for the aesthetics of whatever was left on the street ... I saw with my own eyes the conflict between the obscene profanity and social appearances."

Male colleagues had a slightly easier time trying to understand the basics of the sex trade. The lead editor of this volume, Zunyou Wu, recalls being sent to Yunnan on a similar quest. The HIV specialists in Beijing very much wanted to know whether there was a risk of an epidemic of sexually transmitted HIV following on the heels of the spread of the virus by drug injection. "We asked the head of the local epidemic station to take us to the red light district," recalled Zunyou Wu. "He was shocked and didn't want to take us, but we insisted, and then there we were in these barber shops and beauty parlours that didn't even have any equipment for cutting hair, not a single pair of scissors."

Pretending to be clients, Wu and two colleagues invited sex workers back to their hotel rooms. There, they interviewed the women about their lives and their habits. "They were very offended when they first realised that we didn't want sex. But after we promised to pay, they relaxed and told us many things," Wu said. The "clients" learned that women took antibiotics even when they weren't sick, because they believed that the drugs would protect them against sexually transmitted infections (STIs). They learned that many women also try to ward off infection by using vaginal washes. But most of all, in the course of an evening in which they spoke to six sex workers, they learned that the women who sell sex for a living could be an invaluable resource in helping to plan effective HIV prevention programmes.

The following day, the epidemiologists cast their net wider, inviting the owners of karaoke bars and "beauty parlours" from which sex workers operate to discuss their beliefs and habits. Many of these people are women, and most were initially reluctant to talk to the officials for fear of incriminating themselves. "Then we asked them if their own husbands had ever bought sex and they joked: Well of course. If he's never been to a prostitute, he's not a real man," Zunyou Wu said. Keeping the tone light, the health officials pointed out that that sort of real man could bring diseases home to his wife. After that, the sex establishment owners joined the discussions too. Their contribution helped shape the intervention programmes for sex workers described later in this chapter.

Lessons learned: listening to those you're trying to help

Three decades into the HIV epidemic, it is obvious that the people who are most affected by a problem will be among those best placed to contribute to a solution. But that was not always so apparent. Up until the 1980s, health programming was thought of as the business of professionals. In countries such as China, where the state made a point of trying to provide for the needs of the population, this was even more the case. And yet as public health officials began to learn about the worlds of drug addiction and commercial sex, they realised that they were dealing with a whole different reality.

The more pragmatic researchers quickly understood that they would have to abandon many of the assumptions that had previously underpinned their work. Public health officials the world over tend to assume, for example, that as long as people know about a life-threatening disease and how to prevent it, they will change their behaviour to avoid being infected. But experience in the field quickly showed that wasn't the case. This was a blow for government workers who hoped that their efforts to educate people would be welcomed and acted upon by the local population.

Epidemiologist Susu Liao reflected on her own feelings on finding that villagers in Yunnan were utterly uninterested in learning about AIDS, a disease which was already visibly killing people in their own communities. "This was truly frustrating and seriously crushed our morale. While talking to villagers, we could see how indifferent villagers and even village leaders were about this AIDS disease and even death. Only a few AIDS victims mentioned to us a little about their problems. As each day passed, the glorious glow of our divine mission grew dimmer and dimmer. I could feel that what we thought and what the villagers thought were quite far apart."

This experience led to a very important realisation, one that Liao and her colleagues took forward with them into their future work. "The lessons from Ruili ... reminded me that I need to feel what the people feel and what they really need when I work with them on disease control and prevention. This is perhaps one of the most important truths to remember in the realm of medicine and public health."

This willingness to listen and learn from affected groups is now firmly entrenched in China's response. It is recognised even (or perhaps especially) by policy makers, who tend to live in a more rarefied world, divorced from the situations in which much risk behaviour takes place. Former Vice Minister of Health Longde Wang described his own surprise, much later in the epidemic, at discovering the extent of homosexual activity in China. "When I was abroad, I said there were no gays in China. But sometime later back in China, we began seeing HIV cases in people who were infected through homosexual sex," he said. "So we invited some gay men to a meeting; it was then that I realised some of our thoughts were ridiculous." Initially, public health officials had planned to promote mutual fidelity as the main way of preventing HIV among gay men just as they did among heterosexual communities. "After listening to them in that meeting, we knew that casual sex and multiple partnerships were quite accepted in that community," Longde Wang explained. "So we took a different approach than we did with heterosexuals, and promoted condoms among gay men."

The lesson learned by the earliest field researchers was reinforced. "This experience taught me that to get first-hand information, to really understand the key points of an issue, you have to go to the frontline," the Vice Minister said. "Otherwise all the 'knowledge' of the issue just comes from the imagination, and that's no help at all."

Foreign money opens the door to new approaches

Listening to marginalised groups, respecting their opinions and, indeed, seeing them as part of the solution did not come naturally to many Chinese officials, particularly in the early stages of the epidemic. Indeed it took a little bit of arm-twisting by international organisations that were funding HIV research and prevention programmes to get them on board. In 1996, the World Bank lent China money for HIV prevention. Together with funding from the Australian government, this allowed some entrepreneurial local governments who recognised the threat of HIV to start doing something about it. Shaohua Wang, a former deputy director of the health department in the far western province of Xinjiang, recalled getting funding from the Australian government to start HIV prevention work as early as 1999. "In total, it amounted to about 15 million Australian dollars. This was extremely meaningful for us, not just from a financial standpoint, but also because it brought new experiences, methods and ideas from abroad, in the face of changing social mores in China." These ideas were sorely needed in the westernmost province of Xinjiang, where drug injection had suddenly become quite common, particularly among the majority Uighur population. "The flexibility of the funding was really helpful," Wang said. "Some of the projects were not that expensive, but we were able to engage with a lot of groups and organisations." The funds were especially welcome in Xinjiang, one of the poorest parts of China, where there were many conflicting needs. "There was a lot of stress on the [provincial] government back then, sometimes we couldn't even pay everyone's salaries," Wang remembered. "So trying to find funds for a disease that hadn't yet been deemed a priority was a real challenge."

However, according to epidemiologist Zunyou Wu, now head of NCAIDS, not all local officials were as welcoming of foreign funds, not least because of the bothersome requirement that affected communities should be consulted. "Previously, we thought it was the work of an official to plan programmes, and now we had to involve the target audience in the assessment and in joint planning," he remembered. "There was tremendous resistance." Some officials, especially at the provincial level, simply ignored the requirement that proposed interventions should be focused on high-risk populations, who must first be consulted about what was needed. As a result, many of the initial proposals were rejected. "It was hard to change the philosophy of officials, but if they didn't accept the new way of doing things, they didn't get the money. That was the deal," said Wu. He noted that one of the advantages of accepting money from foreign partners was that it allowed people with different experience and outlook to push for new ways of doing things. "Without that, officials just do what they were already doing."

A subsequent World Bank loan that earmarked funds especially for partnerships with non-governmental organisations provides a good, if accidental, example of the catalytic effect that foreign funding can have. Since there were no health-related groups that were truly independent of government at the time, project officers allowed "GONGOs"– for Government Organised Non-Governmental Organisations– to apply for funds. These included groups such as the Red Cross Society of China and the Women's Federation.

The All-China Women's Federation had, since the 1950s, worked hand in glove with the Communist Party to further the government's agenda as it related to women's affairs. Its stance on issues such as prostitution was therefore necessarily conservative. Though the organisation was, by the mid-1990s, beginning to assert its independence from the government, it was a long way from embracing sex workers' rights. In Fujian province, a deputy director of the federation decided to challenge this position. In her boss's absence, she applied for funds under the World Bank loan project to provide HIV prevention services for sex workers. Her boss, the chairman of the local chapter, was duly enraged; it was not the job of the Women's Federation to help the wicked, she believed. "In her mind, she hated sex workers," recalled a colleague. "The government should just kick ugly things like that out of society, that's what she thought." But the grant was signed and sealed, and she had no choice but to get on with the work. A year later, the chairman admitted to her colleagues that she had been wrong. "She shared this with us: The more contact she had with sex workers, the more she felt [the Women's Federation outreach project] was the right thing to do. First she began to feel sorry for the sex workers. Then, she felt as though they needed help. Finally, she felt like she herself should do something to help them. It was a gradual change. Step by step."

Research is a back door for action

China built up its inventory of HIV prevention interventions bit by bit. Ideas and models developed in other countries, and often witnessed first-hand during study visits, were later adapted to the Chinese situation. During a two-month study tour to Australia, senior public health officials absorbed a key lesson that underpinned everything else they saw: if you want politicians, the public and the holders of the purse strings to support your efforts, it's not enough that an intervention works. Rather, you have to be able to prove that it works.

While some other countries took advantage of a boom in international funding for AIDS prevention by setting up projects right and left without any thought for evaluation, China's small team of AIDS warriors built rigorous measurement of results into a very high proportion of their early intervention efforts. Indeed they often put the focus on measurement very deliberately, as a way of disguising the fact that they were actually providing rather controversial prevention services to the people who needed them. Training sex workers to provide outreach to their colleagues, distributing clean needles to drug injectors, providing methadone to addicts who wanted to quit – all of these services were provided as part of research projects, often run in collaboration with well-known foreign academics. The research aspects of these interventions were not just window-dressing; the programmes were carefully designed to provide robust information. Those data would eventually be essential in allowing the AIDS warriors to make a case for effective interventions on a much larger scale.

One early example involved a programme to promote condom use in Shanghai. Health officials were aware that an aggressive campaign to promote condom use in commercial sex in Thailand had led to a dramatic fall in the number of new sexually transmitted infections, including HIV. Some favoured starting to promote condoms actively in China, but their recommendations were seen as controversial. For many people in authority, condoms were still seen as a badge of wickedness: it was not until 2001 that the Chinese government instructed prosecutors to stop using possession of condoms as evidence to convict individuals suspected of prostitution.

"The condom promotion issue was hotly debated at the time, with the main question being whether it would cause an increase in deviant sexual practices or contribute to the growth of prostitution," remembers Shanghai virologist Laiyi Kang. He decided to find out whether people would use condoms if they were made more readily available. In 1994, with the permission of the Shanghai Bureau of Health and the Public Security Bureau, his team conducted an experiment in a high-end hotel in the city. "We asked the hotel management to place condoms in the bathrooms of all of their guest rooms with a notice that read: 'To avoid pregnancy, sexually transmitted diseases and AIDS, please use a condom.' The next day, we asked the staff to check whether there were used condoms in the trash bins when they cleaned the rooms, keep a record of the number of condoms used and replace them every day." Over four weeks, hotel guests used an average of a quarter of the condoms daily. There were distinct weekly patterns, however, with usage peaking on Saturday nights.

"At first, the hotel had worried that this programme would impact their business, but customers welcomed the programme and some foreign guests even complained that we had only prepared sizes suitable for Chinese guests," recalls Kang. The researcher was pleased with the success of the programme, until he heard from one of his seniors in the Shanghai Bureau of Health that the Public Security Bureau was demanding his arrest. His colleagues, however, defended him; further, they brought the research to the attention of senior decision-makers meeting at the first National Working Forum on the Prevention and Treatment of AIDS. The policies drafted ahead of the forum were largely dogmatic, focusing on efforts to eradicate drug use and commercial sex; there was not any great expectation that these would be altered significantly as a result of the discussions. "After hearing my report, however, representatives agreed unanimously to [also] focus on ... promoting the use of condoms and safe sexual practices." A few years later, Kang met the Public Security Bureau official who had wanted to arrest him. "He came up to me and shook my hand warmly, saying that at the time he didn't realise the importance of my work and that he was truly sorry." As has so often proven the case in China, initially strong differences of opinion regarding effective responses to HIV were resolved through a growing body of grassroots evidence.

A pragmatic response: the customer is always right

Although the Shanghai condom experiment was clearly aimed at preventing HIV, the notice provided with the condoms in hotel rooms mentioned avoiding pregnancy and other STIs. Health bureau staff didn't really care which of these reasons motivated people to use condoms; from the point of view of preventing HIV, the important thing was not *why* people used condoms, it was simply that they *did* use them. It took a while for some people running HIV prevention programmes to realise that success did not depend on making their clients care about AIDS. The trick, rather, was to make their HIV prevention services match whatever it was their clients did care about. Epidemiologist Susu Liao described setting up a clinic providing health information and services for women selling sex along a highway in the holiday island of Hainan in the late 1990s. "The subject matter of the project was AIDS prevention. But we soon realised that AIDS was quite far away from the lives of these girls. To them, this was something new that they'd never seen before. They didn't really care about this problem." Talking to the girls, the researchers realised that what they *did* care about was earning enough money to leave the sex trade. Like most other women, they hoped to get married and have children. The workers at the women's health centre switched their message, emphasising condom use as a way of avoiding sexually transmitted infections that could lead to infertility.

This sort of flexibility – learning on the job – was core to developing intervention models that met the needs of people at highest risk for HIV in China. It was not enough to replicate interventions described in the "Best Practices" documents churned out by international agencies. Researchers and public health workers had to understand the sometimes very different mindset of the people they were trying to serve, to be sensitive to how interventions were perceived, and to adapt accordingly. "The sex workers and shop owners who were from the countryside had a picture of the world quite different from ours," observed Susu Liao. "To them, people who visited the roadside establishment could only be government, police, big boss –that's customers with money to spend – or salesmen. They had this notion of doctors, but only of the kind of doctors who sat in hospitals waiting for patients to come to them. They had never seen, nor could they believe, that doctors from epidemic prevention centres or heath centres went outside for 'disease prevention' and worked free of charge." This made it difficult to establish trust, the researcher said. "They were not happy about us 'outsiders' probing around and seeing the indecent activities going on in their places. This aside, some rejected us also because of the fear that we were trying to do business here or trying to open another place and would soon steal away their customers."

As China's economy continued to boom and leisure industries blossomed, it became increasingly clear that trying to shut down the sex trade did not meet the needs of either sex workers or their clients. "There was a lot of discussion," said China's former Vice Minister of Health, Longde Wang. "Ultimately, we thought that it was not practical to prohibit prostitution as we had done in the early times of the new China, because our economic system had changed. What can you do when you arrest a prostitute in a market economy? Educate her, keep her in custody, and then support her long-term?" Clearly, this would not be feasible. "In a market economy, we need a different approach to spreading knowledge."

To be effective, any approach to working with the sex trade would have to tick a lot of boxes. It had to meet the needs of sex workers and their managers, it had to be acceptable to the local population and politicians, and it had to be affordable. All of this, of course, was on top of its being effective at reducing the risk of HIV transmission. Health officials based in Beijing tried to kick-start experimentation in this area by holding a national training workshop designed to give local health officials and policy makers the skills they needed to set up programmes for sex workers. One of them was epidemiologist Zunyou Wu.

"I remember we held the workshop at the seaside resort of Beihai in Guangxi. It was summertime, so of course there were lots of sex workers on the beach," said Zunyou Wu. After discussing some of their earliest attempts to work with sex workers, the Beijing-based staff set a challenge for the provincial AIDS directors and intervention team leaders attending the workshop. "We gave them homework. We gave each participant 50 Yuan, and told them that the money was to be used to talk to sex workers on the beach. They had to report back the next day about what they had learned." The epidemiologist, who now heads NCAIDS at China CDC, laughed at the memory. "They were all so shocked. The organisers were pushing them into the arms of sex workers. No such training workshop had ever happened in China before!"

The strategy worked, though. Participants came back with all sorts of information. "We learned that some sex workers use double condoms because they think it's stronger, even though in reality it makes the condoms break more easily. They have sex in the sea, in part because they think salt water kills bacteria, but also because they're much less likely to be arrested." Australian sex workers who specialised in teaching their peers how to convince clients to use condoms came and talked at the conference too. The workshop broke new ground, and encouraged many local health bureaus to begin providing services for sex workers.

Research to action: developing workable models in the sex trade

Over time, in small pilot projects in Yunnan, Sichuan and elsewhere in China, an apparently effective model for preventing HIV transmission between female sex workers and their clients emerged. The intervention was based around a "Women's Health Clinic and Counselling Service" which provided screening and treatment for STIs, as well as information about disease prevention and counselling on how to persuade clients to use condoms. Staff based at the clinic would also tour the establishments where most sex was sold, trying to avoid times when women were likely to be with clients. During these visits they provided information and (initially) free condoms, as well as vouchers for clinic visits. Once they had built up a client base, the clinics covered their costs by charging for screening and treatment for sexual infections, and by selling condoms. Both of these services were provided at a discount when compared to the prices charged on the open market.

A formal evaluation of this model was conducted in five cities, none of them in the places where the programme was first developed. Sex workers were asked about their HIV-related knowledge and behaviours, and their use of condoms with clients.

Researchers also tested for two sexually transmitted infections: Chlamydia and gonorrhoea. A year later, going back to the same sites (though not necessarily to the same women) they found that workers reported knowing more, and using condoms more frequently. Importantly, they found that sexually transmitted infections, the surest indicator of possible exposure to a sexually transmitted virus such as HIV, had fallen dramatically. The overall prevalence of gonorrhoea fell from 26% at baseline to 4% after intervention, and the prevalence of Chlamydia fell from about 41 to 26%.[24] Interestingly, only a minority of women (just over a quarter) in the follow-up study said they had visited the health clinics maintained by the project. This may signal that the presence of the clinics improved treatment-seeking from other sources as women shared information with one another and as they all grew more aware of why and how they should avoid infection.

Health officials in China were interested in investigating more than one type of intervention. Simultaneously with the clinic-based model, another intervention for sex workers was tried. Based more closely on Thailand's "100% condom use" programme, it sought to work not with individual sex workers but through the structures of the sex industry, notably the owners of establishments where sex can be bought. Broadly, the idea behind this approach is that the authorities will adopt a more permissive attitude towards illegal activities, such as facilitating commercial sex, in exchange for cooperation in enforcing condom use. This approach requires the active cooperation of the local police, which in China proved problematic at first. In Jingcheng, one of the five cities in which the approach was piloted, the police launched a crackdown on the sex industry just three months into the programme. This was a huge setback; it destroyed all the trust that the health staff had so carefully built up with entertainment industry owners. Though the intervention of local government officials eventually secured the support of the police, the mishap demonstrated that these structural interventions cannot succeed unless the noses of all agencies and levels of government are pointing in the same direction.[25]

An evaluation of the 100% condom programme areas published by the World Health Organization judged this model to be successful. Condom use with the most recent clients rose from between 55 and 60% to around 90% in most sites, according to reports from sex workers. Self-reported behavioural data often raise suspicion:

some people believe that sex workers just tell interviewers what they want to hear. But once again, the reported rise in condom use was corroborated by laboratory data. In Huangpi, syphilis prevalence fell from 8 to 1%, gonorrhoea from 3 to 0% and chlamydia from 30 to 16%. Results from other sites were similarly encouraging.[26]

First, make no enemies

China has come such a long way in addressing HIV and the behaviours that spread it over the last decade that it is easy to forget just how difficult it was to take these early steps towards understanding the epidemic. Trying out different solutions to the sensitive problems spotlighted by that early research was even more fraught with conflict and difficulty. But people who were involved in these early stages of the HIV response in China will not quickly forget the lengths they had to go to, to avoid antagonising officials and communities. Language, for example, was used with great discretion. Clinics that were set up for the sole use of sex workers were called "Women's Health Centres" to avoid drawing unwanted attention to commercial sex. Condoms in hotels were made available ostensibly to avoid pregnancy as well as disease. Programme managers also did their best to avoid too much attention from the press. The four locations chosen for the World Health Organization-sponsored trial of an adapted version of Thailand's 100% condom use programme were all small cities, off the beaten track and far from the gaze of the national media.

The HIV warriors became very skilled at spotting people who might obstruct their work, and trying to win them over. Sometimes they involved potential opponents in foreign study tours so that they might witness successful programmes first hand. On other occasions, they used well-placed allies to demonstrate support from higher up the political chain. Longde Wang, one of the earliest supporters of an active response to HIV in China, became a very important ally once he was appointed Vice Minister of Health. When the government of one badly affected province became nervous about a pilot project for sex workers supported by one of its county governments, HIV officials from Beijing organised a visit to the county for the Vice Minister and other senior officials. One of the officials described the scene: "I accompanied them to the sites, and they talked to sex workers, who told the officials how the intervention had changed their habits and their lives. Now suddenly the local provincial government was very happy and said a lot of good things about their pioneer work."

All of these early interventions were limited in scale, so drew little attention. Despite this, they provided health planners with invaluable information about what works, what doesn't and why. The small group of HIV experts began gradually to swell, growing to include people who were influential in sectors outside health, as well as people who were well placed in the governments of provinces at high risk. None of these projects led to an immediate explosion of activity nationwide, but the AIDS warriors were building up a powerful arsenal of knowledge and experience. They knew these weapons would prove effective when the time was right.

Chapter 4

AIDS Policy: China's Tipping Point

Elizabeth Pisani and Zunyou Wu

"SARS taught us that failing to handle health issues would have a terrible impact on social stability and economic development. It helped us a lot to deal with AIDS transmission."

—Longde Wang, Former Vice Minister of Health

China's pioneering AIDS researchers were not content simply to build up evidence about HIV and the programmes that might prevent its spread. From early on, they worked actively to get the nation's leaders to pay attention to the threat that a widespread HIV epidemic would pose to the country. As early as 1996, an inter-ministerial body called the State Council Coordination Mechanism Committee for AIDS/STD Control and Prevention was created under the chairmanship of Vice Premier Li Lanqing. The State Council is the highest administrative body in China, and the coordinating mechanism was able to bring together 21 ministries, providing each with guidance on its roles and responsibilities, to work on HIV prevention.

Providing guidance, however, was not enough for the scientists: they wanted action. They made their expertise freely available to the State Council's committee, and were rewarded with the publication, in November 1998, of the government's first strategic plan for HIV, which provided a framework for HIV prevention and care through 2010. The long-term plan was remarkable for its pragmatism, steering a careful course so that it remained acceptable to more conservative sectors, such as law enforcement, while allowing for innovative approaches that were already proving successful in small pilot studies. The document also voiced a commitment to learn from other countries:

All the prevention and control work must take the local situation and realities into consideration. The best international practices and experiences will be adapted and put into practice. Prevention and control should be pragmatic, tackling not only the epidemic itself but also its determinants and constraints on anti-epidemic work. It should also be contextualized and make full use of local existing resources...

Preventive measures and methods should be introduced to the general population to make them aware of how they can protect themselves and prevent disease. Education of high-risk groups such as prostitutes and drug abusers about relevant laws and regulations against these activities should aim at behavioral changes in these groups. Condoms should be promoted vigorously and the risk of infection for those sharing needles and syringes for drug injection should be publicized among high-risk populations.[27]

In China, as in most countries, a commitment to bold new policies made on paper does not necessarily translate quickly into real changes on the ground. The AIDS warriors in the scientific community looked for ways to maintain the momentum. They convened a three-day symposium during the 1999 Xiangshan Science Conference, an influential annual gathering supported by the prestigious China Academy of Sciences. As virologist Yi Zeng recalled, the meeting definitely succeeded in waking the scientific community up to the challenges ahead: "Three straight days of discussion and debate showed the seriousness of AIDS from a number of perspectives. The China Academy of Sciences took up the cause, delivering a series of policy recommendations to the State Council."

The scientists' messages promoted greater concern about the possibility of a widespread epidemic at the level of the national government. On 3 April 2000, the State Council held a discussion on the prevention of AIDS and other STIs, and the Politburo met to discuss HIV in early 2001. For the first time, significant domestic funds were put on the table to address the epidemic. Not surprisingly, given the horrific outbreak of HIV among commercial plasma donors five years earlier, the lion's share of the money was earmarked to strengthen the safety of the national blood supply, but national funds were also made available for HIV prevention activities. While that was a very important step forward, the money was not nearly enough to cover the cost of implementing the "China Plan of Action for Containment and Control of HIV/AIDS (2001–2005)", issued by the State Council the same year.

The action plan was spot on epidemiologically: it envisaged necessary programmes including condom promotion, sexual health services for sex workers, opiate substitution therapy and services that helped drug injectors access sterile needles and syringes. Politically, however, it was ahead of its time. Though health officials were broadly supportive of the highly controversial programmes, other ministries and agencies were less convinced, especially in more conservative parts of the country. The plan itself acknowledged this, with a note of frustration. "Some local government leaders are not fully aware of the potential risk of an enlarged HIV epidemic, and the social and economic impact on society in China," the text read. The action plan certainly provided cover for the small, experimental interventions described in Chapter 3, but it quickly became apparent that it lacked the universal political backing necessary to persuade county and provincial governments to implement such sensitive programmes on a vast scale.[28]

The value of international partners

When learning about the behaviours that spread HIV and while trying out different prevention programmes, Chinese scientists and health professionals had discovered the value of working with partners from other countries. They used this strategy politically, too, encouraging high-level representatives from other countries and international organisations to raise the issue of HIV when they visited China.

This became a lot easier after international press reports turned the global spotlight on the "AIDS villages" of central China – areas hollowed out by the epidemic that was triggered by the unsafe blood collection practices described in Chapter 2.

UNAIDS Executive Director Peter Piot, for example, visited Shaanxi, one of the provinces with a significant blood-related HIV outbreak, in November 2001. Speaking the following week at China's first National AIDS & STD Conference, Piot made an impassioned plea for China's leaders to show more resolve in tackling

AIDS. "Over the next two decades what happens in China will determine the global burden of HIV/AIDS," he said. "Whether there will be 10 million people or 50 million people infected in China, that will depend in the first place on whether the country really wakes up on a massive scale...Leadership is what makes the real difference in the fight against AIDS, and leadership from the top."[29]

Less than a year later, in October 2002, United Nations Secretary-General Kofi Annan added his voice to a growing chorus demanding greater commitment from the Chinese leadership. "There is no time to lose if China is to prevent a massive further spread of HIV/AIDS," he told an audience at Zhejiang University. "China is facing a decisive moment."[30]

Cumulatively, these visits did contribute to a gradual change of thinking on behalf of China's policy makers. "Somehow, external voices are always more influential," noted one AIDS programme official. Speeches by foreign officials provided an opportunity for the Chinese media to report on the issue of HIV. But just as importantly, they gave the country's AIDS warriors access to the country's top leadership as Chinese leaders needed to be fully briefed about HIV/AIDS before receiving foreign guests. "We would never have had access to the Premier in normal circumstances," said a Chinese health specialist with extensive experience of trying to interact with politicians.

Foreign dignitaries sometimes influenced China's senior leadership in unplanned ways. Former United States president Bill Clinton told interviewers from the Public Broadcasting Service how he unwittingly forced the first public handshakes between Chinese leaders and an HIV-positive person in November 2003:

I was at Tsinghua University in Beijing, and I gave my speech on AIDS. There were three deputy ministers of the relevant government departments with me at the head table. After I answered a couple of predictable questions, this young man – I later learned he was HIV positive and an activist by the name of Song [Pengfei] – stood up. And you could have been in America: He had, like, a spiky hairdo, and he asked me a really sassy question, and so I said, 'Come up here.' Just on instinct I said, 'Come up here,' because I knew it was being televised nationally. He came

up on the stage, and I put my arm around him and hugged him and shook
his hand, and I took him over and introduced him to the vice ministers.
And the Chinese showed the whole thing on television. They showed this
man, a real person, shaking hands with these government ministers. Within
10 days, the prime minister had 10 AIDS activists in his office. Then before
you knew it, President Hu [Jintao] was out visiting hospitals of people who
were HIV positive ... I knew that the picture could be powerful.[31]

Such events perhaps also underscored in the minds of top Chinese leaders the power
of symbolism in confronting HIV and in chipping away at the stigma encrusted
around the epidemic. It was not enough, they realised, to support evidence-based
HIV policies. They needed to support – and be *seen* to support – the hundreds
of thousands of Chinese citizens who were living with the disease. In late 2004,
Chinese President Hu Jintao said he wanted to meet people with AIDS and asked
his staff to arrange a visit to a Beijing hospital. This was a surprise; normally health
staff have to lobby for months or years to catch the attention of top leaders, let alone
to persuade them to talk to patients. But the President, quite of his own accord, was
determined to meet people with HIV. The visit was arranged for the eve of World
AIDS Day, which falls on 1 December. Shaking hands with patients on the AIDS
wards, Hu promised to help them in every possible way. He made the pledge not just
on his own behalf, he said, but on behalf of all of Chinese society.

Coming to terms with all the numbers

Officials who were keen to do more about HIV in China were still in a bind. On the
one hand, it was clear that prevention and care services couldn't happen on a large
scale without more active leadership from the highest levels of government. On the
other hand, it was very, very difficult to attract that leadership unless they could be
more honest about the scale of the problem. As the plasma donor fiasco underlined,
the default behaviour among Chinese officials faced with a public health crisis at
the turn of the 21st century was denial. Epidemiologists in China's HIV programme
were well aware of this. In the early years of the epidemic, even the official bulletin

of the Chinese Academy of Preventive Medicine's AIDS programme, which carried AIDS case reports and data from other types of HIV surveillance and research, was classified as a confidential internal document.

It was no secret to anyone in China or abroad that statistics produced by government departments were not always accurate due to difficulties in data collection and other problems. This was especially true if they dealt with subjects that might reflect well on local officials (such as economic growth and job creation) or when they might reflect badly (such as uncontrolled outbreaks of infectious disease). The scientists became accustomed to arguing with their more politically minded colleagues in the bureaucracy, urging them to be realistic about the number of people infected with HIV or at risk. Ray Yip, an epidemiologist who headed the China programmes for the US Centers for Disease Control and Prevention and later the Bill and Melinda Gates Foundation, said this required considerable bravery, given bureaucratic cultures rooted in imperial times. "The classic mandarin instinct is to shoot the messenger. If I take bad news to a minister, like AIDS is getting out of hand, they say you must not be doing your job, maybe we should find someone more competent." According to Yip, this was one of the reasons that so little was done following the first investigations into the outbreak of HIV among plasma sellers; it accords with epidemiologist Xiwen Zheng's account, given in Chapter 2, of trying to communicate the results of research honestly. "The scientists were saying we've got a house on fire here, we've got to put it out before the whole village burns down," Yip noted. "But the person who can sound the fire alarm, they don't want to pass that message on to the very top, to the people who can take action."

Suspicion about the validity of any figures published by the government was compounded by an entrenched misunderstanding of what the numbers meant. When interacting with the press, including with foreign journalists, officials usually confined themselves to reporting the number of confirmed, registered HIV cases: 20,711 in September 2000, for example. Officials recognised that this was nothing like the real number of cases; in China as in most other lower- and middle-income countries at the time, only a small fraction of HIV infections had actually been identified through testing.

As early as 1998, when the State Council working group on HIV published the first long-term plan for HIV, it estimated that over 300,000 Chinese citizens had been infected with HIV by the end of 1997. If the epidemic kept growing at its current rate, the document stated, there could be 1.2 million people living with HIV in China by the end of 2000. Though they were published by the highest administrative body in the land, these estimates were not widely publicised. As officials continued to report the number of confirmed HIV cases and journalists continued quite wrongly to assume that this represented the government's official estimate of the total number of people living with HIV in China. This misunderstanding led many people to believe that China was deliberately covering up the extent of its HIV epidemic, even though that was not the case.

Estimating the numbers at risk for HIV: China leads the way

When the outbreaks of HIV fuelled by plasma donation in central China hit the world headlines in late 2000 and early 2001, people began to question China's official HIV data more openly than ever before. This allowed activist health officials to argue for the publication of data-based estimates of the total number of people living with HIV. This made more sense than ever after the Joint United Nations Programme on HIV/AIDS (UNAIDS) published country-specific estimates for the first time in 2000. Using a curve-fitting model, UNAIDS staff in Geneva estimated that half a million Chinese people were living with HIV at the end of 1999. With that number already on public record, China's scientists argued, why not try and do a better job at home? They used a simple spreadsheet-based model that included estimates of the number of drug injectors, sex workers, clients, gay men, and former plasma donors, then combined that information with estimates of the percentage of each of those groups infected with HIV. Using data for the end of 2000, the epidemiologists came up with the figure of 600,000 people living with HIV in China.[32]

Though it was simple, the method was fairly robust. Indeed a similar method was later adopted by the World Health Organization as the recommended method for estimating the number of HIV infections in countries whose epidemics are concentrated in known high-risk groups. This made China a pioneer in the field of

HIV estimation. Using the experience of the first round of estimates coupled with better data sources, the Ministry of Heath updated the figures the following year. In April 2002, they announced that they believed some 850,000 people were living with HIV in the country.

And yet because the estimates were published by the Ministry of Health, everyone questioned their validity.

For the many people who worked hard from the start of the epidemic to really understand what was going on, this disbelief felt like an injustice. The organisations that joined to become the National Centre for AIDS/STD Control & Prevention had sought international guidance in building up a national HIV surveillance system and provided a lot of training and support to provincial governments. Several of the worst affected provinces, led by Yunnan, built up a strong HIV surveillance system in high-risk groups early in the epidemic. Yunnan was also one of the first areas to start systematic surveillance of risk behaviour. Plenty of health officials and others took significant professional risks in arguing to make the most accurate data more widely available, but their efforts did not increase public confidence in official statistics.

UNAIDS rocks the boat

This distrust created a sort of vacuum, which was quickly filled by non-government groups, each with their own sets of statistics. "When you try to hide numbers, well, people will just make them up," said US CDC's Ray Yip. The biggest splash was made by the United Nations Theme Group on HIV/AIDS in China. In June of 2002, just as the international HIV fraternity converged on Barcelona for the biennial AIDS conference and the media were looking for interesting angles on HIV, the Beijing-based Theme Group published a report entitled "HIV/AIDS: China's Titanic Peril".[33] The report was drafted without consulting the Chinese government; it was released at a high-profile press conference in the Chinese capital and was immediately seized upon by the international press. "U.N. Says China Faces AIDS Catastrophe" screamed the headline of the Reuters News Agency report. "U.N. Publicly Chastises China for Inaction on H.I.V. Epidemic" thundered the *New York Times*.[34,35] For several years after the report's publication, virtually all international news coverage of China's epidemic (and many articles in academic journals) quoted the figures in the 'Titanic report' as evidence that China was covering up the extent of its epidemic.

An example comes from a report by global rights advocacy Human Rights Watch on HIV in China: "In December 2002 the Ministry of Health acknowledged one million people living with HIV/AIDS. Other experts have put the number of cases in China higher by varying amounts. A UNAIDS report in China in 2002 estimated as many as 1.5 million people living with HIV/AIDS," the report said.[36] It is ironic, then, that the numbers in what came to be known as "the Titanic report" in fact overlap with Chinese government estimates. The official estimate of 850,000 infections for the end of 2001 was well within the range of 800,000 – 1.5 million infections published in the Titanic report. Though the *New York Times* carefully pointed out the overlap, most press reports simply seized on the number at the high end of the range. Many also enthusiastically drew attention to a prediction that if more were not done to prevent the spread of HIV in China, 10 million people could be infected by 2010. The report incorrectly sourced this figure to the Chinese State Council's own long-term plan of 1998; that document in fact mentioned only that unless action were taken, 1.2 million citizens may be infected by the year 2000. The actual source of the much-quoted projection of up to 10 million infections by 2010 remains unclear to this day.

Other outside bodies made even more extreme predictions. Later in 2002, the United States National Intelligence Council forecast that China would have up to 15 million HIV infections by the end of the decade. "But it was the Titanic report that really hurt," said epidemiologist Zunyou Wu, who was involved in making national HIV estimates at the time the report was published.

It's easy to see why. Here is the dramatic opening to the report:

> *At the dawn of the third millennium, China is on the verge of a catastrophe that could result in unimaginable human suffering, economic loss and social devastation. Indeed, we are now witnessing the unfolding of an HIV/AIDS epidemic of proportions beyond belief... Some of the major factors that have contributed to the relatively slow response to AIDS in China comprise insufficient openness in confronting the epidemic, a lack*

of commitment and leadership at many levels of government, especially provincial and local levels, a lack of adequate resources, a crumbling public health care system, and severe stigma and discrimination against people infected or affected by HIV/AIDS. A potential HIV/AIDS disaster of unimaginable proportion now lies in wait to rattle the country, and it can be feared that in the near future, China might count more HIV infections than any other country in the world.

Coming from the United Nations, which normally tries to tread softly with its larger member states, this was strong stuff indeed.

Bernhard Schwartländer, a co-editor of this volume, headed the group responsible for HIV surveillance and estimation at UNAIDS headquarters in Geneva at the time. He had not known of the report before its publication, and while he thought the estimates it contained were entirely reasonable, he was surprised by the strength of the language. "I remember thinking, oh my God, is that really necessary?" Having supported China in developing its surveillance and estimation systems in the past he was also acutely aware of the different attitudes to statistics. The team in Geneva had been working for some time to develop methods that would allow them to report ranges which would more reliably reflect the uncertainty of estimates that were inevitably based on limited data points. "In a country the size of China, and for a disease like HIV which is mostly invisible and so hard to measure, the difference between 800,000 and 1.5 million is nothing," Schwartländer said."What's important is not the exact number,it's what you are doing about it." But politicians are less comfortable than scientists are with uncertainty. "Especially when there are goals and targets involved, Chinese leaders always want a single number," Schwartländer said. If 1.5 million Chinese citizens were infected with HIV by 2001, then the country couldn't possibly meet the target, laid out in the 1998 long-term plan, of curbing total infections at 1.5 million by the end of 2010. If the true number was closer to the lower end of the range, meeting that target was still possible. "We think of it as reasonable uncertainty. But for a lot of people whose jobs depend on it, the difference between 800,000 and 1.5 million is very concrete."

Although the report caused friction between the Chinese authorities and its partners in the United Nations, both sides now acknowledge that the outcome was broadly positive. "Though it sounded shocking at the time, it's true that the government was very slow to react to the epidemic, especially in the fall-out from the blood donor epidemic," notes Schwartländer. "In retrospect, that report did help to push things forward." Zunyou Wu, now director of NCAIDS at China CDC, agrees: "It was definitely a wake-up call. If you always go slowly and peacefully, you can't change anything."

Former Vice Minister of Health Longde Wang noted that some officials disputed the figures in the Titanic report: "When some experts claimed that the number of people living with HIV/AIDS was close to a million and would approach ten millions in 2010, well, that caused a significant reaction," he said. The most important outcome of the report, he said, was that it encouraged China to collect more reliable data, and to make much more transparent estimates of the epidemic. This process is described at greater length in Chapter 5.

The shock of SARS

By the end of 2002, pressure was clearly building on the Chinese leadership to be more proactive in pushing for the implementation of the existing, highly pragmatic policies around HIV prevention. As the magnitude of the blood-related epidemic in central China began to sink in, more and more voices were also calling for care and treatment to be provided. "There was clearly a feeling that the plasma seller outbreak was the government's fault," said one health official, "that we were at least indirectly responsible for those thousands of infections."

Into this flammable mix, a spark was thrown: Severe Acute Respiratory Syndrome(SARS). SARS is an airborne viral infection that seems to have spread from domestic animals to humans in southern China. The first apparent case was reported to Chinese health authorities in November 2002, but China did not share the information with the World Health Organization until February 2003. During those months of silence, the virus began spreading to other countries. By the time the WHO declared the global outbreak controlled in July 2003, close to 8,300 people had been infected (5,300 of them in mainland China, with another 2,100 in Hong Kong and Taiwan) and 755 had died.

China's failure to confront the SARS epidemic openly and to report cases quickly and honestly in the earlier stage left the country's reputation very badly bruised. But it also opened the door to a new way of doing things. As Human Rights Watch put it in a very strongly worded report:

> *The SARS epidemic has shown both the old face of the Chinese political system, and a potentially new face. Beijing's dark side was exemplified by its initial cover-up of the epidemic, and by its knee-jerk resorting to draconian measures developed during the AIDS epidemic, such as the jailing of 'intentional transmitters.'*

> *But by firing the Minister of Health, the mayor of Beijing, and more than 100 health officials for covering up or under-reporting SARS infection rates, or for not taking prompt and appropriate action, China has established new standards of public accountability.[36]*

Former Vice Minister of Health Longde Wang recognised SARS as a tipping point for greater openness about HIV. "We learned the lesson from the SARS outbreak in 2003," he said. "SARS taught us that failing to handle health issues would have a terrible impact on social stability and economic development. As a result, SARS helped us a lot to deal with HIV transmission." The transition to a more open approach was not easy for everyone. "We did need courage to break down some ingrained ideas, to break through some barriers," the former Vice Minister said. One of those was the idea that news of disease outbreaks would shame China in the eyes of the world. In fact, Longde Wang said, SARS demonstrated that the reverse was true. "China was widely condemned in the international conferences before 2003, [but that changed when] China started to share its experience... You get recognised at home and abroad as long as you take pragmatic action."

The tensions between old and new ways of dealing with disease outbreaks – with some voices encouraging greater openness just as others continued to deny the facts – was confusing for people working on HIV.[36] In the end, advocates of openness won.

One of the important effects of the SARS epidemic was that it removed the bureaucratic filter that usually stood between scientists and the country's most senior politicians. According to US CDC's Ray Yip, "SARS brought the scientists into contact with people they wouldn't normally be able to react with." One of those was Vice Premier Wu Yi. At a meeting called by Wu to discuss SARS in 2003, one of the country's senior virologists, Yi Zeng, had underlined that SARS was relatively easy to control compared to the socially, culturally and politically more complex challenge presented by HIV. Scientists who were at the meeting remember the Vice Premier being struck by the information. Once SARS had been adequately dealt with, she promised, China would take on that more complex challenge. In February 2004, she transformed the earlier coordinating mechanism into the much more vigorous State Council AIDS Working Group, made up of the top figures from 29 ministries and seven provinces.

Less than a year later, in April 2004, the Vice Premier addressed a national conference on HIV. "The present work of HIV/AIDS prevention and control is far from enough," she declared. She called for more accurate estimates of the extent of infection, and more prevention research, as well as a more open and pragmatic attitude. "We must learn the lessons of our success in fighting SARS, and carry out HIV/AIDS prevention and control in a practical, active and urgent way."[37]

A fresh promise of care

Some more cynical observers wondered if the statements the government made in the wake of SARS would have any more effect than the many well-intentioned HIV-related plans that the country has seen since 1998.

One public statement did, however, raise the hopes of even the most cynical. In September 2003, speaking in front of the United Nations General Assembly's special session on HIV/AIDS, Executive Vice Minister of Health Gao Qiang, on behalf of Primer Wen Jiabao, made an extraordinary commitment: the Chinese government promised to provide free antiretroviral treatment for all rural AIDS patients, as well as for poorer patients in China's cities. HIV testing would be made universally available for free to all Chinese citizens via the local CDC or other approved facilities, and all HIV-positive pregnant women would get free antiretroviral drugs and free infant formula milk they needed to reduce transmission of the virus to their babies. On top of that, the state would provide economic support for orphans and families affected by the virus, and free schooling for the children of poor people who were coping with HIV infection.

Gao Qiang had himself previously been a senior official in the Ministry of Finance, so he was acutely aware that these sorts of commitments were meaningless unless they were backed by resources. He convinced relevant ministries and the State Council to put funds aside to pay for the initiative, which was later christened the "Four Frees and One Care" programme. While Gao Qiang lobbied colleagues in other departments to raise domestic spending on health, Gao Qiang also encouraged the judicious use of funds available from other sources. In its earliest incarnation, the Four Frees and One Care programme was underwritten by a grant from the Global Fund to Fight AIDS, Tuberculosis and Malaria. The first grant, of US$90 million, was used largely to provide HIV testing and antiretroviral treatment to people in the seven central provinces of China most affected by the outbreak related to blood-selling. Funding for HIV prevention and care from domestic coffers rose quickly (the details can be seen in Figure 8 of the Appendix). Until 2000 it languished under US$2 million a year. In 2001, with the first five-year plan, that amount rose seven-fold. In 2003 it more than tripled again to almost US$50 million. By 2004, the year when China's leadership really put its weight behind HIV prevention and care, government spending had hit over US$100 million.[38]

These strong signals of greater political commitment were exactly what China's AIDS warriors had been waiting for. As Chapter 3 explained, they had, since the start of the epidemic, been patiently experimenting with different approaches and building up evidence. Now, they apparently had the green light to reproduce their successes on a much larger scale. The story of how they did that is told in Chapter 6. First, however, they took advantage of the opportunity to get a handle on the real scale of the epidemic in China. What they found, described in Chapter 5, took everyone by surprise.

Chapter 5
Finding Those At Risk, China's Way

Zunyou Wu, Elizabeth Pisani and Anuradha Chaddah

"We said, listen, you can't talk about human rights in thin air. Don't HIV-positive people have a right to know their status and get treated? Don't they have a right to prevent transmission to their spouses? Don't the uninfected have the right to not be infected?"

—Zunyou Wu, NCAIDS/China CDC

One of the people who heard Vice Premier Wu Yi's plea for greater openness in the aftermath of the SARS epidemic was Li Keqiang, now China's Premier but at the time the Party Secretary of Henan province. As we saw in Chapter 2, national specialists such as Xiwen Zheng estimated the number of HIV infected plasma sellers in Henan at around 80,000, and activists were claiming ten times as many. However, provincial officials stuck stubbornly to an estimate of 10,000 infections. Backed by the central government's renewed determination to find out the true extent of the epidemic, Li Keqiang encouraged his staff to do whatever was necessary to get to the truth.

Normally, HIV estimates in countries with epidemics similar to China's are made on the basis of data from sentinel surveillance among high-risk groups. In sentinel surveillance, blood is taken from people at high risk for HIV for some therapeutic purpose (such as for syphilis screening and treatment, or assessing patients for drug-related services). The blood is then stripped of personal identifiers and tested for the virus that causes AIDS. That gives health authorities an idea of the overall percentage of people in that risk group who are infected. Applying the percentage to the estimated number of people who share the risk behaviour gives the estimated number of people infected. Of course some people may be infected even though they are not themselves in one of the high-risk groups included in the estimates – the wife of a drug injector, for example, or the husband of a sex worker. Often, information taken from HIV testing among pregnant women is used as a proxy for these secondary infections.

This estimation method is not very well suited, however, to epidemics that were driven by the selling of blood, because most former plasma sellers would not be captured in the sentinel surveillance of high-risk groups. Rather than basing their estimates of the numbers infected on data from sentinel surveillance sites, health officials in Henan and the National Centre for AIDS/STD Control & Prevention took the bold step of trying to find and test all those who might have been put at risk through blood selling. This meant conducting a full door-to-door census and asking every household if anyone in the family had sold blood in the 1990s. Those who said they had indeed sold blood would be offered free HIV testing. Though this would obviously be a huge undertaking, health authorities thought it was the only way to get information good enough to set to rest all the concerns about under-reporting of cases.

More importantly, they realised that if they really were going to deliver on the ambitious commitments made by the country's most senior leaders, and especially on vastly expanding the proportion of people with HIV who would have affordable access to life-prolonging treatment, they would have to have a much better idea of who was infected. Good estimates were needed for planning and monitoring purposes, of course, but to provide people with treatment, health officials needed to know which individuals were infected. Though some voluntary testing services were available in some places, people just weren't using them very much. One study asked participants in a relatively high-prevalence area if they would like to receive more information about HIV, as well as a free HIV test. Vouchers were given to all participants; if they came to the clinic they could claim a small payment whether or not they got tested. Just short of half said that they would like a test, but only one in six turned up at the clinic to claim their payment, and a tiny 3.7% actually took a free HIV test.[39]

Another study that offered confidential HIV testing to couples attending mandatory pre-marital counselling sessions in Anhui province found that only 16%

accepted tests when they were free. When people were charged CNY20 for a test (around US$2.50 at the time), that already low rate plummeted to just 1.4%.[40] The citizens of China's badly affected central provinces, including Anhui, had seen what happened to people who had tested positive for HIV. They were fired from their jobs, rejected by their families and turned away from health services. Discrimination was, as Chapter 8 describes in greater detail, more or less universal. It was hardly surprising, then, that people who suspected they might be at risk were not exactly queuing up to find out whether they were infected.

Activists inside and outside China opposed mass screening of plasma sellers

Their experience mirrored that of countless people around the globe. Since the start of the epidemic, a positive HIV test had exposed individuals to discrimination. And though a handful of studies showed that people who had learned of their infection following a voluntary test took steps to prevent passing on the virus, there was, for the first two and a half decades of the epidemic, very little benefit for individual patients in knowing they were infected. Because of this, both experts and activists in the international HIV world were fiercely wedded to the principle that all testing should be absolutely voluntary and be accompanied by personalised counselling both before and after the test. They also opposed the disclosure of test results to anyone but the client themselves. Since the mid-1990s, when treatment became available to infected people in industrialised countries, the benefit of HIV testing had grown very considerably: if a person tested positive, they could begin to take antiretroviral medicine that could prolong life by years, even decades. But in lower-income countries, this treatment was available only to the most privileged few, while discrimination continued to be experienced by virtually everyone with an HIV diagnosis. Because of this, the international community continued to oppose any sort of mass screening, in China or anywhere else.

Some voices within China shared these concerns. They pointed out that China's successes to date in tackling HIV derived from experiments that learned from what had worked in other countries, and they were reluctant to embark on a programme for which there was no international precedent. They were also sceptical that treatment would be made available to people who tested positive, and they were worried about continuing levels of stigma. Others in China's public health establishment argued forcefully that the potentially massive epidemic of HIV spread by blood-collection practices in central China put the nation in a very different position from other countries. Screening of former blood sellers in central China would achieve two important goals at once, they said. On the one hand, it would provide a much better understanding of the true extent of the blood-driven epidemic. On the other hand, it would allow local governments to identify people who were living with the virus, provide an entry point for treatment, as well as helping them to target important prevention services to help those who were infected, so that they could take measures to reduce the risk of passing the virus on to their spouses, sexual or injecting partners, or infants.

"It was very controversial at the time," said epidemiologist Zunyou Wu, who now heads the China CDC's NCAIDS. He was among those who believed that at least in the seven provinces of central China where the blood trade had been most rampant, a one-time testing of everyone who had sold blood in the mid-1990s was justified. Since the outbreak was not ongoing, a well-implemented screening targeted at the hundreds of thousands of people who sold blood at that time should identify a very substantial proportion of those infected. The government's eventual goal was to provide affordable care and antiretroviral treatment for anyone in China who needed it. But if anyone deserved to be at the front of the queue when it came to free treatment, it was surely the families who had been encouraged to sell their blood to supplement their tiny agricultural earnings. Testing former blood sellers would open the door to treatment for them.

Forging ahead to meet local needs

After much discussion, Henan province took the plunge. Between June and August 2004, the province conducted a door-to-door census, asking whether anyone in the household had sold blood during the mid-1990s. Some 280,300 people said that they had; every one of them was offered a free HIV test. Since individual pretest counselling was judged to be impractical on such a large scale, people were informed of the process of HIV testing and of its benefits through poster and public information campaigns, campaigns that started before the census was even conducted. "The testing campaign was a powerful education tool in its own right, not just for the public, but also for policy makers," observed Wu. "All those hundreds of thousands of tests, it just normalised HIV testing and really reduced stigma. It went beyond the health system; the testing campaign mobilised all of society to participate." The government invested a great deal to arrive at this success, not just politically but also financially, according to former Vice Minister of Health Longde Wang. "Government took many measures to support the screening in the regions: building roads, schools, and wells; setting up clinics and providing free treatment."

Of those who reported having sold blood in the 1990s, 92% agreed to take an HIV test – that's 258,237 tests. Over 23,000 people were identified for the first time as infected with HIV, 9.0% of those tested. In just three months, Henan had identified six times as many newly diagnosed infections as they had reported in the whole of the previous decade. Slightly over half of those were in what are known as "discordant couples", where the infected person has a husband or wife who is not infected. Knowing that they were living with the virus provided these men and women with an important opportunity to avoid passing on the infection within the family. Local health staff provided post-test counselling to those who tested positive, as well as free condoms for those who needed them. They also referred people for the follow-up tests they would need to determine whether they were ready to begin treatment, which at that time was offered to people who had fewer than 200 CD4 cells per millilitre of blood, a measure of a severely compromised immune system. As an expert committee from the Ministry of Health which evaluated the screening reported in 2005: "This type of mass screening could only have been completed in China."[41]

Advocates of the one-time mass screening were surprised by what happened in Henan in the years that followed. "After this campaign, everyone thought there would not be any more HIV-positive tests from plasma [in Henan]," recalled Wu. But each year for the following few years, voluntary testing centres continued to identify several thousand newly diagnosed infections in former plasma sellers. The Ministry of Health expert committee that visited Henan a year after the screening finished found that in the 10 months following the mass screening, over 6,700 former plasma sellers had chosen to have voluntary HIV tests. Some of these may have been from among the 23,000 or so identified blood sellers who refused testing during the mass screening. But it was also clear that a lot of people had refused testing in a more passive way, by simply not reporting that they had sold blood. When they saw that people who tested HIV-positive in the mass screenings were not persecuted, that many did in fact have access to free treatment as promised, they began to come forward of their own accord to the voluntary testing centres set up by the government in many hospitals and clinics.

Zunyou Wu recalled speaking to a woman who was diagnosed with HIV during a voluntary test the year after the mass screening. "She told me that even though she had been a plasma donor, she had lied during the survey. I asked why. Her son was planning to get married in October, she said. So even though she suspected she might be infected, she didn't want to be diagnosed. She worried that if she was diagnosed with HIV, her daughter-in-law would not want to marry her son."

The expert committee found that HIV infection among these late testers was 16.4% – over 80% higher than among those who were tested during the screening. And though the numbers of late testers fell over time, the proportion who tested positive rose. In a careful analysis of data from just four testing sites over the next seven months, a third of over 700 former blood sellers were found to be infected. That suggests that the woman who chatted with Zunyou Wu was not exceptional. People who suspected they might be infected were more likely than others to avoid participating in the screening, but came forward once they saw that they would get financial and healthcare support if they did indeed have HIV. However, the committee reported: "From an analysis of the situation based on data collected through this mass screenings and from discussions with the people involved, the expert group believes that the proportion of former plasma donors who deliberately hid their HIV status is not very high." They estimated that around 15% of people who had actually sold plasma in the outbreak years and who were still alive at the time of the 2004 census denied having sold blood. Interestingly, the four-site study showed that many other people who had not sold plasma but who thought they might have been exposed in other ways also sought out free HIV tests at public services after the screening. Of the people who feared they might be at risk because they had received a blood transfusion, over half were infected with HIV. Some 39% of the men and women who were worried that they may have been infected with HIV through sex also tested positive.

Clearly, there were more former blood sellers living with HIV in Henan than the 23,000 identified in the screening, but probably not stratospherically more. Figures circulated earlier by some activists of "up to a million" infections through this route in Henan were very definitely significant overestimates.[42] It is worth noting, however, that since the outbreak occurred around 1995, many of those infected would have died by the time of the screening a decade later. Without treatment, half of people with otherwise healthy immune systems who contract HIV sexually will have died nine years after they become infected.[43] In poor farming communities where people may have been serially exposed to high infusions of the virus through repeated blood sales and where access to any kind of healthcare is very poor, the proportion who died within a decade of the outbreak would probably have been much higher.

The mass screening among former blood sellers in Henan achieved both of its aims: it improved information about the epidemic and opened the door to treatment for tens of thousands of people who were infected with HIV. With a Herculean effort but in a very short space of time, it provided a robust idea of the extent of the HIV epidemic in the province, putting to rest fears that local authorities were covering up an epidemic. The public, policy makers and healthcare providers all learned a great deal about HIV during the campaign; the stigma that continues to loom over the disease was dented, and many people lost their fear of HIV testing. Most importantly, the screening ratcheted up access to prevention and treatment services for those affected, in part because it identified those in need of care, but also because it motivated service providers to work more effectively. "Our efforts had a good impact in terms of HIV prevention and control, and made the international community change its attitude towards the screening," observed former Vice Minister of Health Longde Wang. Following Henan's success, the Ministry of Health in Beijing encouraged the other provinces that had had an active blood trade to screen all people who had sold plasma there, too. These mass screenings were implemented between October 2004 and June 2005. By the end of June 2005, among 30 provinces, autonomous regions and municipalities excluding Xinjiang, a total of 1,274,046 former plasma sellers had been registered, and 904,746 of them (71%) had been tested for HIV. A total of 25,030 were confirmed HIV-positive, giving an overall HIV prevalence among former plasma sellers of 2.8%.

Taking testing to high risk groups

The second province to take on the challenge of mass screening, Yunnan, was not, in fact, very much affected by blood donation. Yunnan had the oldest and most severe HIV epidemic in China. Driven at first by the sharing of needles between drug injectors, the virus had since spread through the province's active sex industry. Unlike former blood sellers, people who took drugs and sold and bought sex were considered by many to have brought the disease upon themselves. On top of that, the behaviours that had resulted in their contracting HIV were illegal. And, unlike the wave of plasma-driven infections, Yunnan's epidemic was not a one-time outbreak confined to the past. New infections were taking place every day. All of this meant that mass screening in Yunnan posed different challenges compared with in the central provinces of China.

At home and abroad, opponents of targeted mass testing – including those who accepted that the Henan screening experience had been largely positive – once again raised their voices. For one thing, they believed that it would be both impractical and ruinously expensive to repeat the mass testing every year in a situation where HIV may be spreading more or less continuously. But they were also concerned that the screening would be damaging to gay men, sex workers, and above all drug users, exposing them to arrest and increasing the stigma with which they had to cope daily. Public health officials who supported screening all those at high risk, on the other hand, argued that approaches developed in an age before treatment was available, and that prioritised an individual's privacy above all else, were inappropriate in an age of treatment. "The international community was very critical, saying this was a violation of human rights, and of course not international best practice," remembers

Zunyou Wu. He and other colleagues pressed for an approach that took into account the welfare of the uninfected majority as well as those living with HIV. "We said, listen, you can't talk about human rights in thin air. Don't HIV-positive people have a right to know their status and get treated? Don't they have a right to prevent transmission to their spouses? Don't the uninfected have the right to not be infected? When we talk about rights, we need to talk about individual rights, community rights and public rights."

Supporters of more active testing invoked the basic principles of infection control in epidemic outbreaks, including limiting the infectiousness of those who had contracted a disease (either through rapid treatment or, if necessary, by restricting their interaction with people who might be susceptible to infection) and by tracing their contacts. China had used these tactics successfully to shut down the SARS epidemic, and they have been used again more recently to control the Ebola virus in West Africa. But the history of the AIDS epidemic, coming to light as it did among gay men in the United States at a time when homophobia was the norm in that country, had led activists to argue that protecting the right to privacy and non-discrimination of infected individuals was every bit as important as controlling the spread of the virus. "There's a tension between public health and [individual] human rights," conceded Wu. "The way we see it, we feel like there is an obligation to protect the public, especially the uninfected."

Some see the debate as something of a false dichotomy. "We weren't against widespread testing of groups likely to be at risk," recalled Bernhard Schwartländer, a former UNAIDS representative in China. "We were just against mass testing that disrespected privacy." However he recognised that the very concept of privacy differs from one society to another. "In China, if nobody feels that they are lacking privacy, if people don't feel it's a problem, then we shouldn't impose it."

In fact, the advent of effective treatment for HIV had removed some of the tension. This is because the likelihood of passing HIV on to a sexual partner depends in large part on the amount of virus in one's blood or body fluids. Antiretroviral medicines suppress HIV, so people who start on correct treatment early enough in the course of their HIV infection are very, very much less likely to pass infection on to their sex partners than people whose infection remains untreated. In other words, treatment supports the right to a healthy life for people who are living with HIV, while at the same time protecting the public by reducing the spread of the virus. To start on treatment, you have to know you have HIV. And that means taking a test.

At the time that Yunnan started its mass testing of people at high risk for HIV, the international community remained ambivalent about this argument. In July 2004, right in the middle of the mass screening in Henan and with Yunnan already planning its own campaign, UNAIDS and the WHO issued a new policy statement on HIV testing. "UNAIDS/WHO do not support mandatory testing of individuals on public health grounds," the statement said. It did, however, endorse the routine offer of HIV testing in a healthcare setting to people who were at high risk of having been exposed to the virus, as long as follow-up counselling, psycho-social support and treatment were available. The statement did not mention China explicitly, but some paragraphs addressed the concerns raised by the country's approach rather pointedly:

> *The cornerstones of HIV testing scale-up must include improved protection from stigma and discrimination as well as assured access to integrated prevention, treatment and care services. The conditions under which people undergo HIV testing must be anchored in a human rights approach which protects their human rights and pays due respect to ethical principles.*[44]

To many people's surprise, the mass testing in Yunnan in large part complied with most of these principles – though there were exceptions. Over the last three months of 2004, the provincial health authorities identified 424,000 people as being eligible for testing because they were pregnant or at high risk for HIV infection. These included people who were married to or were the child of someone known to have HIV, people who suffered from another sexually transmitted infection or a disease that thrives in people with damaged immune systems, and people whose behaviour exposed them to HIV, principally drug injectors and sex workers. Former plasma sellers were also included on the list. All these people were invited to have a free HIV test, and 98.7% of them agreed – a remarkably high rate which prompted some people to question the "voluntary" nature of the test. Obviously some people, including people in detention or rehabilitation for taking drugs or selling sex, were in no real position to refuse testing.

Overall, 3.2% of those tested were newly discovered to be living with HIV – nearly 13,500 people. In three months, Yunnan had doubled the total number of people diagnosed with HIV in the province since the start of the epidemic. It went on to increase its efforts to make care, treatment and prevention available.

The public health argument had won out. Having followed Yunnan's progress closely, China's central government believed that the benefits of providing a gateway to prevention and care services through testing of groups most likely to have been exposed to the virus far outweighed the risks. In the autumn of 2005, Beijing encouraged all provincial governments to step up their HIV testing efforts, starting by screening high-risk groups. This was one of the first steps in the massive increase in service provision described in greater detail in Chapter 7.

So, how big is the epidemic?

One of the driving forces behind the huge screening efforts of 2004 and 2005 was a desire to understand the magnitude of the epidemic in China which, as Chapter 4 explained, was a subject of considerable debate both nationally and internationally. The near-universal assumption in the pre-SARS age was that Chinese authorities were systematically underestimating the number of people infected with HIV in the country. But no organisation had better data than the Chinese government, and none was able to offer a more reliable picture of what the real figure might be.

By mid-2005, all of China's central provinces had followed Henan's lead and carried out mass screenings of former blood sellers. Most other provinces had emulated Yunnan, and greatly increased testing in the groups most at risk for HIV. This information, added to stepped-up sentinel surveillance, was critical to building up a more accurate picture of the epidemic in this vast and hugely diverse country. The other important component of better estimates, every bit as influential in the final results, was the estimated size of each risk population. By testing a fixed number of people in a given risk population over a couple of weeks once a year, sentinel surveillance systems could provide a fairly robust picture of HIV prevalence for each risk group. For example, a sentinel site for drug users in one county in Yunnan might report that 87 of 200 drug injectors had tested positive for HIV. In other words, HIV prevalence among injectors in that area was 43.5%. Similarly, testing of 200 female sex workers in a market town in Guangdong found only one infection, so prevalence there would be 0.5%. To turn that into an estimate of the total numbers infected, we have to know: 43.5% of *what*? Half a percent of *how many*? In the mid-2000s, only a handful of countries worldwide had made systematic and transparent estimates of the numbers of people in each of the groups that carry an especially high risk of exposure to HIV. China was one of the first.

Beginning in 2003, China CDC had worked together with UNAIDS and several other partners to try to develop and test ways of estimating the number of people in high risk groups. Eventually, they settled on variations on what are known as "multiplier methods". In multiplier methods, you take a known quantity, and then use other data, sometimes from a survey, sometimes from a different, unrelated source, to estimate data that are missing from the original list. It would not be practical, for example, to count every single sex worker in every single establishment in a town. But most towns do have a list of licensed massage parlours, karaoke bars and night clubs, and beauty salons. A "quick and dirty" survey in the town might reveal that 90% of karaoke bars and clubs, 50% of massage parlours and just 15% of beauty parlours are licensed. During the same survey, researchers count the number of women employed at a random sub-set of those establishments, and the number that sell sex. This information can then be applied to the list of licensed premises. First, researchers construct a "complete list", adjusting the number upwards to reflect the missing establishments in each category. Then they multiply the number of establishments by the average number of women selling sex in each type of location. Of course many more sophisticated adjustments can be made, but overall, multiplier methods have now been shown to provide fairly robust estimates of the number of people engaged in high-risk behaviours in many different countries and settings.

Once population size estimates are available, all health staff have to do is apply the HIV prevalence rate for that population to the number of people in the group to get an estimate of the number of people infected. These estimates can of course be made at many levels. A small, relatively homogenous country might make a single estimate for each of the risk groups nationwide. But a country as large and diverse as China must make estimates at much lower administrative levels. In 2005, for the first time, enough data were available to try to make systematic estimates at the level of the prefecture (the highest administrative level after the province). One province, Guangdong, went even further, making separate estimates for each county, then summing them up to get the provincial total.

Past experience suggested that developing estimates was a process that lends itself to disagreement and dispute in every country. Province A does not want to be seen to have more infected people than Province B. Or activists seeking funding for the groups they work with dispute results. "What?! There are three times more gay men infected than drug injectors? That can't be!" These sorts of arguments are most likely to arise when people are faced with the absolute numbers. To protect against this, and to arrive at the most accurate estimates, the group leading the estimation process in 2005 espoused a fundamental principle. They would construct the spreadsheets so that the outputs – the absolute numbers infected – were hidden from participants in the process. Those participants included a wide range of people who had information or experience to contribute to the exercise: among them local health staff, people from the Public Security Bureau, from the department overseeing the entertainment industry, from groups providing prevention and care services to those at risk. All had to agree on two things: the methods, and the input data. Since data combined with method yields result, if they were agreed on those things, no one could later dispute the result if they felt it was too high or too low.

Elizabeth Pisani, a British epidemiologist who worked with the Chinese government in 2005 to support the country's estimation effort on behalf of UNAIDS and WHO, travelled around the country with colleagues from NCAIDS of China CDC, helping provinces to develop their estimates. "There were some very heated debates," she remembers. "People from different institutions had different ideas about which data were most reliable in the local context. Some days, we were still sitting at midnight trying to annotate the spreadsheet to make sure everyone's inputs were recorded." In the end, though, there was always an agreement. "By the end of the process, we were all pretty confident that whatever number came out, it would be as close to the truth as possible with the data we had," she said. "And it was sure as hell going to be more accurate than any previous estimate."

The national figure, when it was finally revealed in an internal meeting at the health ministry in November 2005, came as a surprise. With all the new data at their disposal, and with more rigorous methods than ever before, the epidemiologists had estimated that the total number of people infected with HIV in China at the end of 2005 was 650,000. This put the country's leaders in a quandary. On the one hand, they had just made a huge political commitment to tackling the HIV epidemic honestly and transparently. In other words, they had committed to telling the truth about the magnitude of the epidemic. On the other hand that truth, arrived at using internationally sanctioned methods, showed that the HIV problem was not as severe as had been anticipated. Indeed the estimate was only three-quarters as high as the government's own previous estimate. This was bound to lead to accusations of a cover-up. It did not help that World AIDS Day was approaching fast: everyone in the AIDS world knew that new estimates were underway, and they expected an announcement with great media fanfare on 1 December 1st.

The HIV experts in China CDC argued that the correct results should be made public, just as they had done since the very first outbreak of HIV among drug users in Yunnan in the late 1980s. Knowing that there was likely to be a lot of controversy over the results they prepared for it carefully. "I remember being called in to work on the Sunday morning before World AIDS Day so that we could role-play the press conference and prepare for whatever questions might come up," said epidemiologist Elizabeth Pisani. A former reporter herself, she was assigned the role of the foreign journalist in the mock press conference, asking senior CDC staff difficult questions about government cover-ups.

In the end, the government decided to take a similar tack as it had back in the early days of the Yunnan outbreak. They did release the new estimates, but not until after World AIDS Day, when all the media attention had passed. In the meantime, the ministry held private briefings for academics, HIV support organisations and the staff of UN agencies, explaining the estimation process in exhaustive detail so that misinterpretation would be minimised. Despite this, there were voluble protests, including from AIDS activists such as Yanhai Wan. The National Centre for AIDS/STD Control & Prevention engaged actively with everyone who disputed the figures. "We said here are the methods, here are the data, you tell us what's wrong," said one official who worked on the estimates. "No one could find fault." Quickly, the objections melted away.

Manageable goals

The estimates were lower than expected for a good reason. HIV sentinel surveillance systems tend to be set up first in populations and in areas of greatest risk. This means that they tend to portray the "worst case" scenario. The prevalence rates measured in the worst-affected places then get applied to make estimates over a wide geographical area, simply because no other data are available. As the HIV surveillance system becomes more comprehensive, with sites established over a greater variety of areas, data provide a better approximation of reality. This pattern applies all over the world.Indeed in 2007, UNAIDS revised its estimates of the number of people living with HIV worldwide down from 40 million to 33 million for largely the same reasons – the geographical expansion of surveillance systems showed that there was more variation in the epidemic than previously thought.[45]

China, huge and socially and economically diverse, is more affected by this sort of variation than most countries. The current surveillance system shows that just a fifth of the country's 303 sentinel sites for drug injectors record HIV prevalence of higher than 5%, almost all of them in the west and south-west of the country. Of over 500 surveillance sites among sex workers, just 7% record rates of infection above 1%. Those sites, fewer than 40 in all, are similarly concentrated in the south-western areas of the country where surveillance was first well established. Because of the massive nationwide testing efforts of 2004 and 2005, the 2005 estimates could for the first time take this variability into account.

As confidence grew that the new estimates were the best possible reflection of reality, health authorities at the national and at provincial and county levels faced a new challenge. With a solid idea of how many people were infected with HIV, they had no alternative but to start planning to provide care and treatment for those that needed it. Similarly, the more robust estimates of the numbers of people in groups at high risk for infection underlined the need for a huge scale-up in prevention services for those who were not yet infected – the overwhelming majority, in every risk group. The next chapter describes how China rose to that challenge.

Chapter 6

Fulfilling a Promise: Universal Care

Zunyou Wu and Elizabeth Pisani

"Hesitation should be avoided. We must be practical, realistic and open-minded."

—Former Vice Premier Wu Yi

Even before the extent of the epidemic became more reliably known, China's leaders had signalled their renewed determination to tackle HIV in all of its dimensions, social and economic as well as medical. Because dedicated health officials and researchers had been running pilot programmes and building up evidence for well over a decade, there was a lot of information available about which approaches might work best. But most of these approaches went against the grain for many of the local politicians and senior bureaucrats who would have to implement them across the nation.

Former Vice Minister of Health Longde Wang told a story that illustrates some of the early obstacles to getting local leaders on board. At a conference, the Vice Minister ran into a professor from the Communist Party Central Committee's training academy. "He told us that the Vice President of Party School prohibited staff from giving trainees information about HIV/AIDS prevention." The Vice Minister thought this was a lost opportunity to create long-term political support for the fight against AIDS. "If leaders and cadres understood the significance of HIV/AIDS control and prevention, it would be easy to promote interventions in the areas where they governed," he said. The Vice Minister and his staff made an appointment to meet the vice president of the academy. They pointed out the seriousness with which national leaders viewed HIV/AIDS. "We said it was inappropriate to forbid the distribution of an AIDS booklet in Party School."Not only did the academy vice president accept their argument, he went further than the Vice Minister had hoped. He invited the Ministry of Health to provide not just booklets, but lectures on HIV/AIDS for all party cadres attending the academy. The Vice Minister seized the opportunity. "At the same time, I suggested running a nationwide audio-visual education programme to allow more leaders and cadres in our country to learn these lessons." The video-training, conducted in June 2006, was a great success, attended by some120,000 government officials. "The situation turned upside down after the lecture," the Vice Minister noted.

However, he stressed that this sort of initiation for politicians and senior civil servants had to be institutionalised and firmly embedded in regular leadership. "In our [increasingly decentralised] administrative system, there's a high turnover of leaders. A leader might be supportive of HIV-related work, but when he or she leaves, it's not by any means certain that their replacement will understand its importance," Wang said. He told the story of a city mayor who removed an AIDS prevention billboard that his predecessor had erected near the central railway station. "He thought that the publicity would have a negative effect on the image of the city."

As Chapter 4 mentioned, a frank and impassioned speech by Vice Premier Wu Yi to the revamped State Council HIV/AIDS Working Committee in July 2004 provided both the permission and the motivation to move forward on a large scale with the unorthodox approaches that had been tried out by the AIDS warriors in the earlier years of the epidemic. The Vice Premier reminded colleagues that the epidemic related to blood collection was firmly under control, leaving the country to deal with epidemics driven by sex and drug injection, as well as the transmission of HIV from mother to infant. She noted that some interventions in these areas had worked, mentioning specifically condom promotion, needle exchange and methadone maintenance. "But these are only limited pilot experiments" she said. She recognised that they remained controversial in some quarters: "People have different views about them; there are still obstacles in understanding and more work needs to be done around implementation. But hesitation should be avoided. We must be practical, realistic and open-minded. These effective interventions must be firmly put into practice to prevent the further spreading of [the] HIV/AIDS epidemic."

Here it was, then, a clarion call from the highest level of government to scale up controversial but effective programmes. Immediately, the HIV specialists in the Ministry of Health grabbed the opportunity they had been working toward for so long. The remainder of this chapter describes the successes and continuing challenges China faced in its first phase of rapid programme scale-up.

HIV testing as a gateway to care

The least controversial area for HIV programmers was providing treatment to those infected with the virus. This was almost universally regarded as desirable, at least in areas where many people had become infected by selling or receiving blood. It was also the central commitment of the high profile "Four Frees and One Care" policy. Though, as discussed in Chapter 5, HIV testing can sometimes generate debate, it is unquestionably an entry point for care. In 2004, slightly fewer than 20 million HIV tests were carried out in China. These included antenatal testing for pregnant women, as well as all of the tests undertaken in the targeted mass screenings that year. While the number seems vast, the data shown in Figure 9 in the Appendix show that it was to rise quite steadily to more than seven times that number by 2015.

In 2005, after the larger screenings of higher-risk groups were over, close to 41,000 HIV infections were newly identified during 25.3 million tests, a positive-to-test ratio of 0.16%. Ten years later 143.6 million HIV tests were performed, and over 115,000 infections were identified for the first time; though the ratio of newly identified cases to tests halved, the number of cases identified rose by 143%. The number of places where people could go to get a test rocketed also. In 2007, there were fewer than 3,700 testing sites, many of them funded by external organisations to provide voluntary counselling and testing services. By 2015, over 24,700 sites provided testing, one third of them to individuals who sought out tests voluntarily. The other tests happened in hospital and clinic settings, or in places where people at high risk gather. Details of who was tested for HIV in 2015 are given in Table 1 in the Appendix.

Recently, a trial was conducted to see whether HIV testing could effectively be offered as a routine part of service provision in community health centres, which provide the bulk of primary care in China. By selecting patients who were likely to be at risk, the primary health services detected more cases per test than hospitals did. But in some areas, there is still resistance from care providers to integrating HIV testing into routine primary healthcare. HIV testing adds to their workload, the follow-on services for care and treatment are not always easy to access at the community level, and discrimination remains rife. Some worry that patients will be put off seeking treatment for other conditions if they know they'll be tested for HIV.[46] "The will of the mass is not same as the expert's will, but it is also worthy of respect," observed one Chinese doctor involved with HIV testing policy.

China's latest HIV estimates, made with much the same methods as those used in 2005, put the number of people living with HIV in China at 850,000 in 2015. By the end of 2015, 577,423 people had been reported as having confirmed HIV infection since the start of the epidemic, not including 182,882 reported to have died of AIDS. In other words, about 68% of those believed to be currently living with HIV in China have been identified. To go in less than a decade from a state of overwhelming denial to one where more than 60% of those who might need care have been identified is no small achievement.

One thing continues to perplex health officials, however. With the extraordinary scale-up of testing, and especially with efforts to encourage those most likely to be at risk for HIV to come forward for regular tests, authorities expected that they would over time identify people in need of care much earlier in the course of their infection. As we explain below, that's important because earlier diagnosis leads to more effective treatment. Doctors estimate the progression of untreated infections by counting a patient's CD4 blood cells to determine how badly compromised their immune system is. Thinking massive targeted testing would mean earlier diagnosis, they expected to see CD4 count at first diagnosis rise. In fact, however, it has remained stubbornly low in some groups. People infected heterosexually are especially likely to present late for testing, perhaps because they do not feel at risk, and are less likely to be targeted by public health or outreach programmes than other groups such as drug injectors, sex workers, or men who have sex with men.

In an effort to open the door to treatment for even more of the people who need it, Chinese health officials have thus pioneered another intervention that some consider unorthodox: the active tracing and testing of regular and casual sex partners of newly diagnosed individuals. For years contact tracing, as this practice is known, had been considered taboo in the international HIV community; people feared that it would expose the infected partner to blame, rejection or violence. China began contact tracing in the central provinces where most people had been infected while selling plasma, a behaviour that was not frowned upon by society. They judged that offering infected partners treatment and protecting HIV-negative partners from becoming infected was justification enough for actively encouraging people to disclose their status and bring their partners for testing. When the policy was first actively promoted in 2006, the regular sex partners of around 35% people with newly confirmed diagnoses were followed up for testing. By 2012, an astonishing 90% of the spouses or live-in partners of infected heterosexuals had been tested and knew their own HIV status. Those that test HIV-negative are actively encouraged to repeat the testing every year.

The rocky road to treatment

A positive HIV screening test is just the first of several steps towards HIV treatment. Though antiretroviral treatment was also provided free from 2004 under the "Four Frees and One Care" programme, patients had to find money to pay for up to eleven other laboratory tests before they could qualify for free treatment. The costs varied a great deal by region: one study measured them at less than US$30 in some sites, over US$150 in others.[47] National protocols required any patient with a positive result on their screening test to come back later and give blood for further testing. About a third of patients never bothered to come back.[48] Blood samples for those who did come back were sent for another screening test at a higher-level laboratory; if that test was positive the result was confirmed by a test known as a Western Blot, which is expensive and complicated to perform. It could take up to a month to go through all the steps required just to get a confirmed HIV diagnosis; in that time health staff sometimes lost contact with patients even before they could be referred to the next stage, the CD4 test. Here was another opportunity for potential patients to be lost to the system. In 2006, at the start of the treatment scale-up, just 20% of those with confirmed HIV diagnoses (and only 13% of those who had initially screened HIV-positive) went on to get a CD4 count within six months. In that time, their immune systems suffered further damage, which diminished the prospect for successful treatment. A careful analysis of the national database showed that 9% of people newly diagnosed with HIV between 2006 and 2012 died within six months. Seven out of ten of them never got a CD4 test, so couldn't access the medicines that might have saved their lives.[49] Figure 11 in the Appendix shows how dramatically that has changed.

CD4 tests are important because they give doctors a good indication of how well a patient's immune system is functioning. CD4 cells are an important part of a healthy immune system, defending the body from other infections. A healthy adult will normally have somewhere between 500 and 1,200 CD4 cells per millilitre of blood. But HIV attacks those cells, so that over time there are fewer and fewer left, and the body is therefore less and less able to defend itself against disease. When the CD4 cell count falls below 200 or so, people begin to suffer from things that would normally be fought off by the immune system. In the context of HIV infection, these are known as opportunistic infections: they are one of the defining characteristics of the syndrome known as AIDS. An analysis of treatment and survival among those diagnosed in the earlier years of the expansion of China's treatment programme (until 2009) found that CD4 count at diagnosis was exceptionally important in explaining who lived and who died. People who had a CD4 count of between 50 and 199 were twice as likely to die over a given year as those with higher CD4 counts (even though the sicker people were also 2.6 times more likely to be taking antiretroviral treatment). People whose first diagnosis did not come until their CD4 cells were reduced to fewer than 50 per millilitre were between five and six times more likely to die.

This analysis added to a growing body of evidence from around the world showing that sooner was better as far as treatment was concerned. When China first started to scale up HIV treatment, it offered free antiretroviral medicine to anyone whose CD4 count was below 200. That was in line with common practice in lower-income countries at the time. But with new evidence of the strong link between early treatment and survival, China's policymakers changed the rules. From 2008, anyone whose CD4 cell count was below 350 cells per millilitre of blood became eligible for treatment. In 2006, 47% of people qualified for treatment at their first CD4 test. The remainder were asked to come back for tests every six months until they fell below that threshold. With the change in rules, a total of 61% of confirmed cases qualified for medication. That added 5,000 people to those eligible for treatment just among that year's diagnoses. The treatment threshold was raised again in 2014, so that anyone with CD4 counts below 500 – the lower limit of the normal range – could access free antiretrovirals if they met the other residence and income requirements. Finally, in February of 2016, the government announced it would get rid of the CD4 threshold entirely: anyone with a confirmed HIV diagnosis can seek treatment immediately.

Getting medicine to those who need it

Despite repeatedly expanding the pool of people eligible for treatment, China managed to increase not just the number of people on treatment but also treatment "coverage"– the proportion of people who qualify for antiretroviral medications who are actually getting them. In 2005, fewer than one in 10 of the Chinese citizens who had tested eligible for treatment were receiving antiretrovirals. As Figure 12 in the Appendix shows, by 2015 it was closer to 9 in 10. In large part because more and more people could get life-saving treatment, the death rate among people with HIV infection plummeted, from 18% a year in 2005 to below 4% in 2015.

The country enrolled close to 108,000 new patients on treatment in 2015, over 12 times as many as were enrolled just eight years earlier. (For comparison, the number of new patients starting treatment in China in 2015 was about 25% higher than the total number of people ever on treatment in the United Kingdom.) In total, over 387,000 people were receiving antiretroviral treatment in China in 2015.

The sharp rise in treatment, in terms both of coverage and of raw numbers, is an unprecedented success by any measure. However some public health officials were dissatisfied that every year, over 50,000 people who were known to be eligible for treatment were not getting it. They also knew that the real number in need was higher: the stubbornly low CD4 counts at first test showed that most people were still not coming for testing until they had been infected for several years. And when people did come for testing, the drop-out rate between initial screening and entry into care was unacceptably high. That was clearly leading to unnecessary deaths. Overall, 64% of the 21,000 people with a confirmed HIV diagnosis who died in China in 2013 did not survive long enough to begin treatment, and over a third never even got a CD4 count.

In response to this, health officials experimented in two counties with a "one-stop shop" system for diagnosis and entry into HIV care. Between 2010 and 2014, they consolidated the four separate steps previously taken by prospective patients between HIV screening and HIV treatment down to just one. Any person who screened positive at any site in the study area was given an appointment at the local county hospital the following Wednesday. At that hospital visit, blood for confirmatory and CD4 tests was drawn and the patient underwent a physical exam by a doctor trained in AIDS care. The doctor prescribed immediate treatment for opportunistic infections if needed. Results of the blood tests were returned to the county hospital within 48 hours: hospital staff were incentivised to follow up with all patients in need of care. The results were dramatic. The time between a first positive screening test and initiation on antiretrovirals for those that needed them was roughly two months using the standard system. The "one-stop shop" system brought that down to less than two weeks. Under the old system, fewer than 40% of people with a confirmed HIV infection ever even started taking antiretroviral medicines, and more than one in four died within a year. With the "one-stop shop", 90% of newly diagnosed people who met the threshold were given medicines, and just one in ten of all those diagnosed died within a year.[50]

It would doubtless be a logistic challenge to provide these one-stop testing and treatment services in all of the 4,226 health facilities across the 2,415 counties of China that are currently providing antiretroviral medicines for those that need them. But the progress that China has made so far in providing treatment on a massive scale, and the dedication of public health officials to trying new things to improve services for users, suggest that the country will rise to this challenge more quickly than many would have thought possible just a decade ago.

Making treatment work for patients, and doctors

Of course getting people on to antiretroviral treatment is not the end of the story. HIV medicines only work if they are taken correctly and consistently. Even then, patients can develop resistance or react badly to particular medicines in the 'cocktail' that makes up the treatment regimen. Often, patients need support to help them follow their treatment regime. "Treatment is not just pills, it's an approach," explained Bernhard Schwartländer, a physician and former UNAIDS representative who now heads the World Health Organization office in China. "To get sustained viral suppression, the system needs to work for the patient; you need adherence support, and simplified regimens." That means, for example, giving patients medicines that combine several different active ingredients in one pill, so that they do not have to remember to take several different pills at different times of the day. Combined formulations of pills, often known as "fixed-dose combinations", have been available on the international market since 1997, but they are not licensed for sale in China. Public health authorities in China would like to see that change.

The early focus on provision of antiretroviral medicine eclipsed another area that some argue is equally important: the treatment of the opportunistic infections that feed on a weakened immune system. If people wait until they feel unwell to present for testing, it is likely that they are already suffering from one or more of these other infections when they are first diagnosed with HIV. Unless these infections are treated quickly, patients could die of tuberculosis, pneumonia or other illnesses before the antiretroviral medicine has a chance to get to work suppressing HIV and restoring the immune system.

Most opportunistic infections are cheaper to treat than HIV. But, especially in the early years of the "Four Frees and One Care" programme, the cost of treating secondary diseases was not automatically covered by the government. In 2004, the Ministries of Health and Finance directed local governments to pay for the treatment of opportunistic infections for those patients who could not afford it, but this instruction was implemented very unevenly. In 2005 and 2006, an international charity working in two provinces recorded what patients would have had to pay out of their own pockets if they weren't sponsored by the NGO. They showed that the expense of treating other infections ranged between US$140 and US$400 a year for patients who did not need hospitalisation, and between US$1,200 and US$4,000 a year for patients with complex diseases that required advanced hospital care.[47] Since then, efforts have been made to expand free or subsidised treatment of other diseases associated with HIV. But former Vice Minister of Health LongdeWang said much remains to be done. Speaking a decade after that study was undertaken, he said: "The rate of antiretroviral treatment will not be increased without treating opportunistic infections." The reason for this is partly embedded in the incentives through which hospitals and doctors get paid. Historically, Chinese hospitals (and by extension doctors) have derived a significant portion of their income by selling drugs to patients. By introducing free HIV treatment, the government cut off a potentially important source of income. HIV is the most stigmatised infection in China, so health professionals were already reluctant to work with AIDS patients; removing the added income that they might earn from drug sales (by making antiretrovirals free) further reduced the enthusiasm of many doctors for treating these patients.

One way for a hospital to reduce the number of HIV-related patients it had to deal with was to refuse those patients care because they could not afford to pay to be treated for the associated opportunistic infections, which were not always covered by public programmes. "HIV/AIDS cases, most of whom were very poor, went to medical institutions for free treatment. However, the medical institutions still have to support the [rest of the infrastructure of care] because only 3–5% [of the associated cost of care] was subsidised by government," explained Wang. "HIV/AIDS patients get free antiretroviral treatment in hospital. But, besides HIV, they also contract opportunistic infections, for which there is no free treatment policy. The patients may not be able to afford the treatment. Hence, not every patient can be accepted to get treatment in hospital."The Vice Minister believed that free treatment should be systematically expanded to include opportunistic infections: "The government should pick up the cost of both of these types of treatment. Because it is not only a personal issue; it also relates to the transmission of an infectious disease." But he suggested that more action would be needed to resolve the problem of disincentives to treat HIV patients on the part of hospitals. "Maybe we can solve the problem through medical and health service reform," he said.

Certainly, there are still challenges to be met in increasing the proportion of people who learn of their HIV infection soon after it occurs, and in optimising treatment. So far, however, things are headed in the right direction: the number of infections identified continues to rise faster than estimates of new infection; the proportion of people with identified HIV infection in need of treatment who receive antiretrovirals continues to increase, and the death rate among both treated and untreated patients has fallen markedly.

Preventing HIV transmission from mother to infant

Among HIV prevention programmes, just one has developed with relatively little controversy: the programme that aims to help pregnant women to avoid passing the HIV virus on to their newborn children, often referred to by the initials PMTCT, for "prevention of mother to child transmission". HIV-infected women can pass the virus on to their infants during pregnancy, during the process of childbirth itself, and during breastfeeding. Efforts to prevent this transmission start with HIV testing for pregnant women, ideally early in their pregnancy. Those identified as HIV-positive should be treated with antiretroviral drugs. In addition, the newborn infant is treated with the drugs for a short period, to reduce susceptibility if they are indeed exposed to the virus.

China ramped up its PMTCT programme very quickly. In 2004, only a tiny handful of pilot projects were testing pregnant women for HIV. The national programme began in 2005; by 2015, over 88 million pregnant women had been screened for HIV infection, 19 million of them in 2015 alone – or 81% of all women who were known to be pregnant in China that year. Around one in 10,000 of those women was found to be infected with HIV. A surprisingly high proportion – over half in one city-wide study over an 11 year period – did not carry the pregnancy to term. Of those who did, however, very high proportions were given antiretroviral medication for both themselves and their infants. In the early years of the programme, most of the testing took place once the woman was already in labour, but over time that proportion has dropped dramatically. By 2011, eight out of ten women identified with HIV because of their pregnancy in China were being started on antiretroviral treatment during antenatal care. The programme has contributed to a 52% fall in the rate of HIV transmission from mother to child between 2005 and 2014, from 12.8% to 6.1%.

Keeping drug users safe from HIV

It was one thing to invest public money to protect newborns from an incurable virus. But politically and socially, it was quite another thing to spend money on health services for adults who voluntarily took illegal and toxic substances in order to get high. Indeed HIV prevention and care services for drug injectors have been more difficult to implement than programmes for any other risk group in most countries around the world. For more than two decades, no central government funds were spent on clean injecting equipment for drug injectors in the United States because of opposition from conservative politicians. The Thai government, much praised for its pragmatic approach to HIV prevention in the sex trade, failed to reduce infection rates among drug users. To this day, infections continue to spread rapidly through shared needles in some parts of Eastern Europe. And all of this despite the fact that a few brave countries – first Scotland and then the rest of the United Kingdom, as well as Australia and the Netherlands – had shown that ensuring easy access to sterile injecting equipment for drug injectors was one of the most effective, and cost-effective, HIV prevention approaches available.

Things were no different in China. Under the guise of research, the hard-working scientists described in Chapter 3 had, in fact, begun to experiment with approaches that they had witnessed in Australia and elsewhere, including needle exchange and methadone maintenance. Seeing the opportunity presented by the greater openness that followed the SARS epidemic, they rushed to present their early findings to senior policymakers, inviting them also to visit intervention sites. China's Premier, Wen Jiabao, was one of the earliest leaders to appeal for sympathetic treatment of drug users. Former Vice Minister of Health Longde Wang also reported being touched by his visits to drug users. "Young people addicted to drugs tended to be smart and sociable, and very curious," he observed. Noting that relapse rates were typically above 90% (and having met one drug user who was in a compulsory detoxification camp for the 18th time), he believed other approaches were necessary. "In an open, market-based economy, drug use can't be controlled only depending on anti-drug movements or compulsory detoxification," said Wang. "[In Yunnan] I held discussions with the local police, and I noted that these young people did deserve to be rescued."

In pushing for a more pragmatic approach, however, the Chinese government had to be careful not to alienate more conservative colleagues, especially those in the security forces who had spent long years trying to keep the threat of drugs at bay with more traditional tactics focusing on prohibition. In her seminal speech of 2004, Vice Premier Wu Yi described the delicate path that the country must tread. She recognised that the two behaviours thought to be driving HIV in China at the time – drug injection and commercial sex – were illegal, and that reducing the incidence of the behaviours could also reduce the spread of HIV. But she called for pragmatism. "These phenomena are hard to uproot immediately, and may persist for a considerable time. So we must combine prevention and crack-down together to deal with these persistent ailments of society." Specifically mentioning successful pilot projects providing clean needles and methadone to drug injectors, Wu Yi appealed to people with different viewpoints to work together. "Each district and department concerned must apply these intervention measures in a practical and rational way; must fully understand that necessary intervention measures and the crack-down on illegal behaviours share the same fundamental aim. They must stoutly and actively implement interventions, using as a standard of success whether it promotes HIV/ AIDS prevention and control, and whether it helps maintain people's health and security."

In other words, the nation's leaders were putting health concerns ahead of ideological warfare against behaviours that were considered socially undesirable. The Vice Premier reiterated this important message in a ground-breaking teleconference in November 2005, during which she addressed some 200,000 officials from across the country, including people working at the county level, where authorities were sometimes resistant to new ideas and approaches. A health official who witnessed the call described its tone. "Essentially, what she said to people was: Listen; if you understand what we are doing and why we are doing it, that's great. If you don't understand, that's fine too, as long as you do it. You can worry about understanding it later," the official said.

Even though the nation's most senior leaders repeatedly made known their absolute determination to tackle HIV pragmatically, there were still pockets of resistance, especially from security forces. Many believed that making clean needles and syringes available to drug injectors made it look as though the government supported illegal drug use. Methadone programmes, which give addicts syrup or pills that mimic some of the effects of heroin, seemed even worse to some people – like using public money to buy drugs for people who didn't want to quit. They found it difficult to suddenly start thinking of drug addiction as an illness, not a crime. In the end it was data, as much as politics, that led to their eventual support for effective HIV prevention for drug injectors. The small projects experimenting with making needles cheaply and easily available had reported significant success in reducing new HIV infections, as did the methadone maintenance programmes. But the eight official pilot projects testing out methadone presented some other very interesting results as well. When drug injectors were recruited into the methadone programmes, 21% of them admitted to having been involved in crime – theft, drug dealing etc. After joining the programme, they no longer had to buy heroin every day to feed their drug habit. That meant that they no longer needed as much cash. Self-reported crime rates plummeted by four-fifths, to under 4%. The job security of drug users improved too, as did their relationship with their families.[51] In addition, they grew in confidence. A health official who accompanied Vice Minister of Health Longde Wang on a visit to a methadone clinic described the interaction between the minister and one of the clinic's clients. "This drug user, he was on methadone, and he was chatting very happily to the minister. He said: 'For the first time in my adult life, I feel like a human being. I can even look a policeman in the eye. Before I always used to be ashamed and run away.'"

When the Public Security Bureau (PSB) checked with their own records, they found that crime rates had indeed fallen in the areas around the methadone pilot programmes, and the local drug markets also appeared to have shrunk. Even those police officers who were not much interested in the health and welfare of individual drug users were happy to see less petty crime and less drug dealing. "Involving the security services was a complete game-changer," said Bernhard Schwartländer, who worked for UNAIDS at the time. "Once there was a framework for harm reduction the PSB just got on with it."

"Getting on with it" happened very quickly indeed once the decision had been made to expand methadone services for drug injectors in parts of the country where heroin use was most common. Even health officials who had been pushing for an expansion of these clearly successful services were taken aback. Zunyou Wu, who was involved in evaluating the pilot programmes, remembers being asked by the Ministry of Health to get 305 clinics up and running in a matter of months. "I said it's just not possible, we need to buy so many things, you need to have safety monitoring, it takes a lot of time to set up a clinic." It took over a year to set up the first 101 clinics. But the pressure was on, and the team was gaining experience. "We opened the next 204 methadone maintenance clinics in just 50 days." Zunyou Wu shook his head at the memory of those frenzied times. New clinics have been opened every year since then; by the end of 2015, there were 785 methadone clinics in operation, including 29 mobile vans. These full service sites support another 325 satellite sites. Since 2011, these sites have been providing services to around 200,000 heroin users a year. The number of clients has fallen slightly since a peak in 2012; at the end of 2015, some 170,000 former injectors were regular clients of methadone services. For those who stay in the programme – about eight in ten clients each year – methadone maintenance is certainly working well. Newly identified HIV infections over a year fell from one person in every 105 clients in 2006 to one in 500 by 2012, and further to one in 1,000 by 2015.

Needle and syringe programmes have also expanded quickly over time. They tend to be provided in areas where there are not quite so many injectors – methadone maintenance services require more infrastructure and medical oversight, and are thus more cost-effective in areas where many heroin injectors are concentrated in a relatively small geographical area. The very first trial needle and syringe programmes began in the early 2000s, and the number has expanded dramatically since 2005. They are sometimes run by community groups and were until recently often funded by overseas partners, so the number of active sites fluctuates more than the more institutionalised methadone maintenance services. Over the last few years, around 900 sites have been providing services to an average of around 42,000 drug injectors every month.

Despite growing support from many sectors, it is not always easy to keep clients safe; recently, for example, the police in some areas have been arresting clients of methadone programmes if they suspect they are simultaneously using heroin. Overall, however, methadone and safe-injecting programmes have contributed to a steep fall in the proportion of drug users shown to be HIV-infected in nationwide sentinel surveillance. Prevalence in this group has fallen by over half since the programmes were first introduced in earnest in 2005, from 7.5% to 3.6%. While some of this reduction will be because infected drug users had difficulty accessing HIV treatment and thus died, a great deal of it will be because methadone and safe-injecting programmes are effectively protecting these citizens from becoming infected.

Clients of both types of programmes report being pleased with the services they receive. Health officials have, however, spotted opportunities for further improvement. Prevention services still reach only a minority of the people believed to inject drugs in China; more could be done to help get services to those who need them by helping drug users in one setting access services in another. One example is testing and notification. In line with guidance from the State Council, efforts to reduce drug use through detoxification continue in parallel with services that prioritise disease prevention. Though relapse is, in practice, the norm after compulsory detoxification, rehabilitation centres rarely refer patients to methadone maintenance services on release. HIV testing for drug users in detention and in compulsory detoxification centres continues to be routine, but not all people who test positive are routinely told of their HIV infection, meaning that they can't access care. It also means their sex partners and children, who may also need care, will not be referred for HIV testing. Analysis of the national treatment database shows that people infected during drug injection were just half as likely to be on antiretroviral treatment compared with former blood sellers by 2009; they were also much less likely to be treated compared with people infected sexually.[52] When drug users who are in contact with state services of any sort – both health- and security-related – are provided with counselling, HIV testing and referral for prevention and care services as appropriate, China will more rapidly reach the national goal of minimising the spread of HIV and the damage it causes to individuals and society.

Preventing HIV transmission between men and women during sex

Early in the HIV epidemic in China, health officials worried that the virus would spread from people who injected drugs to their sex partners. Especially worrying, from the point of view of a national epidemic, was the fact that around a quarter of male injectors reported in the earliest behavioural surveys that they regularly bought sex from women. Though there were relatively few female injectors, close to half of those that were surveyed said they supported their drug habit by selling sex.[22] By the late 1990s it was clear to everyone that the sex trade had returned to China with a vengeance. Prostitution was especially active in border areas where men gathered in order to visit casinos in neighbouring countries – precisely the areas where the cross-border trade in heroin had already kick-started the spread of HIV.

As Chapter 3 described, public health officials, researchers and even organisations such as the Women's Federation had tried out several different approaches to controlling the spread of HIV through commercial sex in the earliest years of the epidemic. When the nation's top leadership turned its attention to controlling HIV, it recognised these efforts. Vice Premier Wu Yi noted that the trial of the "100% Condom Use" approach promoted by the World Health Organization had worked well. "Actively popularising the use of condoms, we should dispense condoms for free or install condom vending machines in public places where high-risk populations are concentrated," she declared. More than a decade later, this hardly sounds radical. But in 2004, when China's obscenity laws still prohibited condom advertising, it was a big step.

The Ministry of Health was keen to do more to promote condom use in commercial sex. But they had to think carefully about how best to do it, bearing in mind that some colleagues still saw prostitution primarily as a crime that should be stamped out by the police. Former Vice Minister of Health Longde Wang recalled the discussions at the time: "Who would be chosen to do the dissemination and education? We thought [local] health departments were not suitable for this work." The fear was, in part, that politicians who ran health services locally might not support efforts to extend services to sex workers. Instead, the Ministry of Health proposed that epidemic prevention stations, the frontline of a public health service that was still relatively centralised, be trained to take on the task of HIV prevention in high-risk groups. They formed teams known as "Gao Gan", which in Chinese sounds the same as "senior cadre". Forming these special teams was a bold move, but necessary, according to the Vice Minister. "At that time, gay men were under the surface of the water. So the target beneficiaries for our teams work were female sex workers. They worked mainly at night, while we were off duty in the evening. How could we get in touch with the sex workers? That was why we built teams that worked in the evening."

Once the decision was made, things once again moved quickly. Within a year, with funding provided by the central government, close to 2,700 teams were in place around the country, most of them with between six and twelve members.[53]"There were over 20,000 staff in all," said Longde Wang, "all doing outreach for sex workers in entertainment venues. We didn't try to stop the work on which the sex workers depended to support their families. But we told them that they were at high risk of getting infected with AIDS and other sexually transmitted diseases. Once you were infected with HIV, how would you be able to support your family?" The Vice Minister observed that the approach was not without its challenges, particularly in securing the support of public security. But by taking education to the bars and massage parlours, health staff were able to give HIV-related information to over 600,000 sex workers each month.

The active outreach programmes were reported to reach nine out of ten sex workers by 2015, with seven out of ten being tested for HIV annually. These outreach programmes are very likely to have contributed to the low prevalence of HIV among female sex workers in China. Across the country as a whole, around one sex worker out of every 500 is infected with HIV, compared with one in 20 in several other Asian countries. Infections are clustered in the west and south-west of China, and careful analysis of study results shows that a high proportion of infected sex workers are also drug injectors.[54] A recent review of 583 studies of condom use by female sex workers in China reported that the proportion of sex workers using condoms with their most recent client rose from 54% in 2000 to 85% in 2011.[55] Although condom use with non-paying partners also rose, the increase was more limited, and some studies have reported persistently high rates of other sexually transmitted infections over the same period.

Though the proportion of sex workers reached by HIV prevention programmes grew by over four-fifths between 2007 and 2013, the proportion who said that they had had an HIV test and received the results of it within the last year grew by just over a third, remaining at 38%. That, and continuing infection with curable STIs, suggests that there is still room for expansion in the services offered to sex workers. Treating those sexual infections that can be cured is important to limit their spread and the damage they can do to a woman's health, including her ability to bear children. But it is also critical to HIV control, because people who have other, untreated infections are more likely to pass HIV on to others if they are infected with the virus, and more likely to become infected with it if they are uninfected but exposed.

When China started attacking HIV transmission on a large scale in 2004, it was aware that people who were already infected could easily pass HIV on to their regular sex partners if that partner was uninfected (in the medical jargon, if the couple had discordant HIV status). This prompted the proactive finding and testing of partners described earlier. Because treatment lowers the amount of virus in body fluids and thus makes people with HIV less infectious, the government also ignored CD4 count restrictions for HIV-positive people whose spouse was uninfected. The infected person in a discordant couple was able to access treatment whether or not they met the treatment criteria. On top of that, discordant couples were given intensive prevention counselling and free condoms. In badly affected provinces, doctors have to show that they are supporting discordant couples in preventing onward transmission as a condition for getting their medical licences renewed.

As the programme expanded, the number of couples known to be discordant grew each year. By 2015, the number had reached 110,000, up from 59,000 in 2010. At the start of that period, only 45% of the infected partners in those couples were on treatment. By 2015 that proportion had risen to 78%. In 2015, the Chinese government reported that the proportion of regular partners of heterosexuals living with HIV who acquired infection in a given year had dropped by nearly two-thirds over the previous four years, from 2.6% to 1.0%.

Early in the epidemic, the overwhelming majority of women infected heterosexually reported being infected by their husbands, while most men reported contracting HIV in commercial sex. That has shifted over time, as Figure 6 and other data in the Appendix show. Now, much higher proportions of both men and women report that their heterosexually acquired infection happened during sex with a casual partner. Casual relationships are much more diffuse than commercial sex; it is much more difficult to devise effective (and cost-effective) prevention strategies for this setting than it is for commercial sex.

Another shift in sexual behaviour that poses similar challenges for HIV prevention in China is the apparent increase in sex between men. Chapter 7 will describe just how big this change has been.

Hitting the target

China may once have been criticised for being slow to react appropriately to the threat of HIV, but there's no question that it has made up for any early lapses. Observers in other countries have marvelled at the scale of the response and the speed with which it was achieved once political leadership was firmly in place. What, they ask, is the secret to providing so many services to so many people so quickly?

The answers include a dedicated public health workforce with very consistent leadership that had, as Chapter 3 described, been building up experience for some years. But a good portion of the success may be attributed to the judicious use of well-chosen targets. China has always been fond of setting targets to guide performance. In the past, people setting the targets have not always thought very carefully about the effects they might have: encouraging misreporting of statistics, for example, or forcing workers to neglect important tasks which are not driven by targets in order to achieve those that are. That led to a certain amount of trial and error in all areas of government. As former Vice Minister of Health Longde Wang described, HIV was no exception. He pointed to the very first months during which methadone maintenance services were being piloted in eight clinics in 2004. "In the months after the clinics were set up, there was actually a gradual decrease in the number of drug users [coming for methadone]," he said. This was surprising: "Many drug users were very poor and had to commit crimes to get money to buy drugs. Now they could spend just five to ten Renminbi [CNY5–10] per day to get methadone. So why did the numbers go down? Later, primary level medical staff told us that the local plain-clothes police waited at the entrance of the clinic and arrested the clients who came for methadone." It turned out that the police had targets of their own. "Because of their work targets, local police had to arrest a certain number of drug users every month and put them into compulsory detoxification institutions. It was easy for the police to find drug users at the methadone clinics," the Vice Minister said.

It goes without saying that drug injectors were not going to use services that landed them in jail. Active dialogue with a fellow Vice Minister responsible for public security saved the day. Once senior officers realised that the incentive structures for PSB officers might stand in the way of protecting the Chinese public against HIV, things changed. "After the discussion, the Ministry of Public Security supported methadone clinics," recounted Longde Wang. "He even set the quarterly number of clients who attended the clinics as an evaluation of performance for local police." It was a useful reminder of both the dangers and the advantages of setting targets.

Targets were first formally used to support the scale up of HIV services in 2006, when they were set to encourage treatment. Zunyou Wu had at the time just taken over as director of NCAIDS. "I decided to use targets for treatment because treatment is much more predictable than prevention," he said. That's mostly because there is a clear denominator: the number of people with confirmed HIV infection.

China CDC set targets for new HIV diagnoses as well, encouraging staff to focus their testing services among the people most likely to have an undiagnosed HIV infection. The idea of targets was not universally welcomed. "At the time, there was huge resistance from some of our colleagues," Wu said. But the Centre went ahead with target setting, framing them as incentives. Those who failed to meet targets got a small payment; those who met them got a bonus.

In 2011, the Centre hoped to see 75,000 new diagnoses, with 40,000 patients newly enrolled on antiretroviral treatment. Health service providers came up just a fraction short on diagnoses, registering 74,517 newly confirmed cases, but exceeded the treatment target by over 5,000 people, or 14%. As health services get better at providing treatment, the targets have become more demanding: 100,000 new diagnoses in 2015, and 90,000 people newly initiated on treatment. Still, hardworking staff continue to exceed targets, by 15% on new diagnoses and 20% on patients newly enrolled on treatment.

Targets, which also help with service planning, are now set across a range of verifiable indicators. Some fear this will eventually encourage misreporting, but experience so far suggests that when targets are kept realistic, they can help motivate service providers to go the extra mile. They have helped China to reach a huge number of people with essential prevention and care services in a few short years. By 2015, the country was well on the way to meeting the ambitious goals it set for itself in 2004. But the challenges in the next phase of the response, discussed in Chapter 7, will require even more innovation.

China Takes Charge of a Changing Epidemic

Zunyou Wu and Elizabeth Pisani

"We said to them: you are supporting China; that means you need to support our national needs... Donors can be very strong-minded, but we are even stronger minded."

—Zunyou Wu, Director, NCAIDS

When the AIDS warriors in China's academies and health institutions started experimenting with responses to the epidemic, their efforts were largely funded with foreign money. UN agencies; the international development wing of the governments of Australia, the United Kingdom, the United States and other nations; multilateral organisations such as the Global Fund to Fight AIDS, Tuberculosis and Malaria; private charities such as the Ford Foundation and the Bill and Melinda Gates Foundation – all of these provided support for HIV prevention and/or treatment activities in China. The Chinese government's contribution to the response rose dramatically following the "tipping point" described in Chapter 4. But even then, most of the original funding for provision of treatment to people in areas with epidemics driven by plasma sales was provided by the Global Fund.

As noted in Chapter 3, China benefited a great deal from partnership with foreign donors and lenders. But there were downsides, too. Donors tended to have their own priorities, ones that didn't necessarily match China's needs. Especially in the early years their support sometimes overlapped – popular causes or locations got more funding than they needed, while some important issues were left wanting. Most importantly, though, they all had different reporting requirements, and they rarely shared the information they collected. This made it hard for the government to keep track of service provision or to plan effectively, because they didn't always know who was doing how much of what, where and for whom. For health officials at the local level the different reporting requirements were a nightmare. Here's an account related by Elizabeth Pisani, an epidemiologist who worked with China CDC to develop national estimates of the size of populations at risk for HIV in 2005:

> *Wang [not his real name] had been pulled out of Dali to be trained in how to estimate the number of prostitutes locally, and he was quite cross about it. He'd already counted prostitutes in Dali three times in the previous year, he said. Once for the China–UK prevention programme, once for a US-funded programme and once for the Chinese government. Now he was being asked to do it again with Global Fund money. 'Count, count, count. And no money for prevention.' Wang was getting louder as he got more worked up. I could see why he was upset. 'Why don't you just give all the donors the same count and have done with it?' I asked. Wang looked shocked. 'But they've all given me money to count!' he bellowed. 'If I didn't count for each of them, that would be corruption!'[56]*

Local health workers found themselves filling the same data into different forms over and over. Sometimes, the very same donor required data in more than one format, depending on the year the project was approved. The forms demanded by the Chinese government were different again. "It was driving everyone crazy," remarked NCAIDS director Zunyou Wu. It is entirely understandable that funders should want to know how the money they provide is being spent. Rigorous monitoring of what a programme spends and what it achieves is necessary to make sure that programmes are being run efficiently; reporting achievements also helps increase public support for continued funding. But people running HIV programmes shouldn't have to spend more time and funds monitoring what they do than doing it.

The fragmentation was not a problem exclusive to foreign funders. Even within China CDC, information related to HIV programmes was held in eight different databases. Databases for sentinel surveillance, case reporting, treatment, prevention, methadone provision and other indicators were often run by different divisions; there was no easy way of looking at the big picture.

A single, integrated data system

In 2006, NCAIDS decided that everyone would benefit from a single, integrated data platform designed primarily to meet national needs. The first order of business was to decide which data would be included. It was a mammoth task. Two senior staff worked full time collecting and reviewing all of the monitoring and evaluation forms and standardised indicators used for data collection and reporting by government agencies and by foreign-funded projects. They then held a series of consultations and workshops to agree on a single set of indicators and reporting forms. The process took two full years, and entailed a lot of argument. "Some of the foreign projects, they complained a lot. Each donor lobbied to have their own indicators, complaining that they would not be able to show accountability," recalled Zunyou Wu. "We said to them: you are supporting China; that means you need to support our national needs. If you don't want to support our integrated system, then you can just quit." The NCAIDS Director chuckled. "No one quit. Donors can be very strong-minded. But we are even stronger minded." China was also in a relatively strong position because by the time the system was launched in 2008, the Chinese government already provided the majority of funding for HIV prevention and care in the country. "It's harder for other countries to do, because they have to respect their donors' requirements."

The system, known as Comprehensive Response Information Management System (CRIMS), provides a single, web-based portal which allows programme managers to see what is going on in the national epidemic in real time. It provides simple web-based data entry forms which minimise data management requirements, and provides standardised statistical reports which allow for at-a-glance analysis of trends. The platform was developed by a private contractor at the cost of some CNY400,000 (around US$55,000); maintenance costs about the same again each year. Highly secure, it allows data for everyone diagnosed as HIV-positive in China to be entered at patient level, including their CD4 test results and treatment status. Patients on methadone can also be tracked at the individual level. Other data such as use of prevention services are reported in aggregate by site.

The system greatly simplifies the once torturous task of reporting on internationally mandated targets such as the Millennium Development Goals, designed to measure progress in human health and welfare. Far more importantly, however, it provides programme managers with an easy way of spotting possible problem areas in the HIV epidemic and the response, so that they can quickly take necessary action. "Once we implemented it, everyone stopped complaining," observed Wu, who directed the project.

The value of the system became apparent almost immediately. Three early examples highlight the different ways in which it proved useful. In the first example, the system was used to spot an unrecognised area of very high prevalence. Data from a voluntary HIV testing site in Liangshan prefecture in the south-western province of Sichuan reported that over a third of all clients were testing positive. In the old reporting system, staff in Beijing would probably have assumed a typo, or an error in transcription as the data got sent through paper records and by e-mail from testing site to county office, from county to prefecture and on up through the chain. In the new system, there is little room for such errors. CRIMS allowed staff in Beijing easily to check other data from the same site (data that would previously have been in a different database held by a different division). Sure enough, the data for HIV prevalence among women in the same county who were routinely tested during pregnancy were also very high: between 2.6% and 5.1% at different sites, compared with a national average of just 0.2%. China CDC staff in Beijing then contacted local staff to organise a population-based survey. They tested some 31,100 villagers in one county, an area with a large ethnic minority population, and found that 7.0% of general public aged 15–60 were living with HIV. Much of the infection was linked to drug injection. The central and provincial governments quickly committed extra manpower and funds to help the remote prefecture step up prevention and cope with high levels of infection. Furthermore Premier Wen Jiabao spent World AIDS Day 2010 in Liangshan.

Ironically, Liangshan was one of the sites in which a UK-funded HIV prevention programme had been operating for some years. The project's activities included supporting local data collection, so the high levels of risk and infection should have been no surprise. "There may have been good data, but no one paid attention," said Zunyou Wu. "It belonged to whoever collected it; everyone owned their own bit." With the CRIMS system, data from every source go into a single integrated system that is scanned daily by four full-time staff in China CDC in Beijing.

CDC staff at other levels also have access to all the data for their own areas, but they do not always have the skilled manpower to track the data and analyse their implications. This was perhaps the case in the second example of the early use of CRIMS, this time to spot problems with the treatment programme. The province of Guangxi, bordering Vietnam, has a busy sex trade and a fair number of heroin users; it was one of the earliest provinces to develop an indigenous HIV epidemic driven by risk behaviour and by the time the CRIMS system became active, many people in Guangxi needed treatment. Staff in Beijing had for some time been under the impression that Guangxi was rolling out their treatment programme quite effectively. "But then we looked at the data pulled together in CRIMS and we saw that they had unexpectedly high mortality. The CD4 data suggested the epidemic was really horrible, and so many people were dying without ever getting any treatment," said Zunyou Wu. "They had the highest case fatality in the country." Staff from Beijing went to discuss their observations with provincial officials. "When we showed them the data their faces just went ashen." The exchange led to a huge leap in political commitment from provincial leaders, and thus in resources. Guangxi is now the only province in China which has a deputy director in the health bureau dedicated entirely to responding to HIV.

CRIMS has also come into its own as a prevention monitoring tool. The third example of quick-fire use of the system comes from methadone clinics, which report consumption of the opiate substitute as well individual client visit data. In a quick analysis which calculated average consumption per client and compared averages across clinics, the data from a single site in the southern province of Guangdong leapt out at CDC staff. The clinic was consistently consuming much more methadone than was justified by its client load. A site visit and investigation quickly established that clinic staff had been illegally selling methadone on the black market. CRIMS is not just a health database, it seems; it's also a tool for spotting misconduct.

The evolving epidemic

The CRIMS system has helped Chinese officials and others to see "the big picture" of the epidemic. Many people, especially those who have worked for many years at the local and provincial levels, now perceive shifts in the epidemic that require shifts in the response. One major shift is in the epidemiology, in who is getting infected. But there is also a shift in time horizons, and in perceptions about what strategies are needed in the face of new challenges.

Shaohua Wang, Deputy Director of Xinjiang Health Department, summarises these shifts. "In the early stages of the epidemic in China, HIV prevention and control took on the appearance of acute infectious disease management," he said. At the time, it was a necessary response. "If we hadn't done that, we wouldn't have got to where we are today. But it was hard on resources and unsuitable for the long term." His description of the initial fire-fighting approach was echoed by Guohui Wu, the Director of CDC's AIDS division in Chongqing city. "I remember when I began to work on AIDS it resembled more of a disaster response, a state of emergency. We would address issues as they came up, and made plans as we went along." That has changed. "Now we have a stronger infrastructure and better regulatory controls." He and others are happy to take a more structured, longer-term view. "This is not a short-term battle, we have to think of it as a long-term war," observed Lin Lu, Director of Yunnan CDC.

But it is not just the time horizon that needs to shift. People who have been on-the-ground observers of the evolving epidemic observe that in fighting a long-term war, great generals avoid fighting the same battle over and over again. China has been winning battles one by one: first, infections through poor blood donation practices were virtually eradicated. Then, effective prevention among drug injectors brought the rate of new HIV infections in that group right down. Condom promotion and treatment of other sexually transmitted infections among female sex workers prevented the virus from ever taking off in commercial sex in China. Most recently, treatment services have been extended to most of the people that need them.

105

Inevitably, the spotlight now turns to the challenges that remain.

Most observers of China's response to HIV, and indeed many of the actors in that response, are full of praise for what has been achieved, but they note that most of the effective prevention strategies so far have centred on biomedical service provision. Some find it frustrating that these biomedical successes have not, by themselves, been enough to shut down the epidemic. Guohui Wu, the microbiologist who now heads the AIDS division in Chongqing CDC, expressed this disappointment: "With other outbreaks, I can isolate the bacteria, use the right antibiotics, and a week later the epidemic is controlled and there is a great sense of accomplishment in my heart. But with HIV/AIDS, we work very hard, but still we keep discovering new infections. This perplexes me: why is there still so much infection?... Do people not know they are at risk? They do know, so how with that knowledge do they still get infected?" This frustration sometimes takes a personal toll: "When I look at old photographs, when I was a manager in the microbiology department and had less stress, I had a lot more hair!" the doctor said ruefully.

A socially embedded disease requires social responses

The realisation that new infections continue despite the best efforts of health authorities has led many to argue that it is now time for an approach that does more to shape the social and cultural contexts which contribute to risky behaviour and which stand in the way of specialised prevention and care services.

"AIDS is not only a medical disease, but also a social problem," said Xi Chen, Deputy Director of Hunan provinces CDC. "If we take a social and psychological approach as well as a biological one, HIV prevention will go better." Xiping Huan, head of the AIDS Division in Jiangsu CDC, absolutely agrees. "We prevention people are a little bit like scavengers on the waterfront. We run about, salvaging what we can when the tide comes in, with the foam. But why are the waves producing foam like that? As a society, we need to think about that. Family upbringing, social relations, why someone engages in risky sex – this disease is driven by more than just a pathogen."

As pointed out in Chapter 1, HIVs pathway into China and its early spread were facilitated by the sweeping social changes that came with the Open Door policy. Now China is undergoing another wave of social change. In common with the rest of the world, China is seeing traditional ways of communicating, of building relationships and of doing business disrupted by technology. The country has also experienced nearly three decades of rapid economic growth – millions have been catapulted out of poverty and into a consumerist society in which traditional collectivist values are less esteemed than disposable income.

Jiangsu CDC's Xiping Huan puts it succinctly. "The country is awash in drugs, new and old. Social media and all these new dating apps – these new platforms emerge just at a time when the economy is booming and people are beginning to assert their individuality. We need to think forward about these things, because they will allow AIDS to develop in different ways."

Community organisations working in HIV agree wholeheartedly. But they point out that however much they would like to, the health authorities now tasked with controlling HIV have no clear way of taking a more socially embedded approach. "There has been a huge amount of progress over the last decade or more; we absolutely have to recognise that," said Lin Meng, who heads the China Alliance of People Living with HIV/AIDS (CAP+). "It's not wrong that the government takes care of the biomedical side of the epidemic. But we currently need to deal with social and cultural aspects as well. The government knows this perfectly well. They know that HIV is a rights issue, that they also need to respond culturally, politically structurally. But if they admit this, who will do what's necessary? Whose responsibility is it? A change in approach would require the health sector to give a lot of resources and authority to other people..." With a shrug, the activist let the sentence trail off.

Gay men on the frontlines

Jiangsu CDC's Xiping Huan was quite right when she pointed out that social media, drugs, ready cash and a desire for self-expression "will allow AIDS to develop in different ways". In fact, it is already happening. In the decade and a half since infection through plasma sales was halted, the HIV epidemic in China has shifted from being an epidemic driven by drug injection to one dominated by infections transmitted in sex between men. Just 10 years ago, in 2006, 1.4% of gay men included in sentinel surveillance tested positive for HIV. That's about one out of every 70 gay men tested. Figure 2 in the Appendix shows that by 2015, that fraction had risen to 8% – around one in 12.

In sheer numbers of newly identified cases, gay men have traded places with drug injectors. In 2011, about the same number of cases were newly identified in both populations – 10,570 among drug users, and 10,917 among gay men. Newly identified infections in drug users have fallen every year since then, while among gay men they have risen every year, as illustrated in Figure 3 of the Appendix. By 2015, newly identified infections among drug injectors had fallen by more than half, to just over 5,000. Among men infected via sex with other men, on the other hand, the number of newly identified infections more than tripled, to over 32,600. These infections are not concentrated in China's west and south-west, the site of the epidemics driven by drug injection and commercial sex. However, the gay epidemic is different: high rates of infection are springing up in big cities all over China. Finally, three decades into the course of HIV in China, the country has the epidemic it originally anticipated, way back in the mid-1980s when the first cases of AIDS were identified.

Homosexuality is far from unknown in Chinese culture – it is frequently depicted in classical art, and described in many novels of the imperial era – and it is not illegal. However, the modern Chinese state has little tolerance for same-sex relations, and families frown on the behaviour in part because it stands in the way of procreation and the continuation of the family line, which remains all-important in Chinese culture. Le Geng, the founder and CEO of BlueD (pronounced "blue dee"), China's biggest gay dating app, explained the attitudes of different groups. "The government disapproves of homosexuality because they associate it with corrupted Western values," he said. "And ordinary people disapprove because of the carrying on the family line thing." He himself has experienced both sorts of disapproval. He had to leave his job as a policeman after his sexual preference was made public in an internet video. "As for my family, they're very supportive of what I'm doing in a business sense, but they're not so happy on the personal level."

One of the effects of this social disapproval is probably that estimates become skewed. As the Appendix describes in greater detail, the proportion of men reporting being infected heterosexually is suspiciously high compared with the proportion of women who are infected. Anecdotal evidence suggests that many men infected through sex with another man don't want to admit it. Ray Yip, formerly the head of a US CDC-supported HIV programme in Beijing, tells of a day when he was invited out by a community group that works in HIV prevention. "We were up near the Great Wall, it was a nice hot day, and I was hiking with a group of ten guys, all of them HIV-positive. I asked each and every one of them about what they reported when they got diagnosed, and not one of them, when they did their first epidemiological intake form, 'fessed up' to being gay. They all said they had sex with a [female] sex worker, only once." Yet every one of these men was in fact infected via anal sex with another man. China CDC has done its own assessment of the accuracy of initial risk reporting, and estimates that about 15% of gay men misreport their route of infection.

The fear of social disapproval affects more than just the statistics. For many years it acted as a strong brake on sexual relations between men in China just as it did in Western countries. That fear was eroded fairly slowly in the West, beginning in the 1970s in large cities. There, the braver gay men would gather in bars, clubs, saunas and even specific parks to meet one another. For the first time, it was relatively easy to identify potential sex partners; it was no coincidence that the HIV epidemic followed rather quickly on this small social opening, and in this limited circle.

The very same social opening that allowed people to exchange sex partners and spread HIV also provided the platform for an effective response. In the face of government indifference, gay men in the United States gathered together to face the crisis their own community was suffering. Activists went to the very venues where people were looking for sex partners. They began educating, entreating, persuading, even shaming their peers into using condoms when having sex. The owners of gay bars and saunas participated actively in these efforts. Since this same community was watching its members die, month after month, year after year, it was not hard to develop a sense of shared responsibility and accountability. In San Francisco, the epicentre of the epidemic, condom use during anal sex between men rose from zero to 70% between 1982 and 1985, and new infections began to fall.

China's social opening, however, has happened at a very different time. Two factors in particular mean that the shape of the HIV epidemic among gay men in this country will look different to that in the West. The first is technology. As Xiping Huan suggested, social networking apps have changed the face of sexual risk, not just in China but the world over. Apps such as Grindr and Hornet allow men in many countries to find potential sex partners without having to go to a bar where they might be seen by a family member or work colleague, without having to suffer the sometimes excruciating embarrassment of the face-to-face meeting. In 2015, Grindr had some 6 million monthly users worldwide, including in China. BlueD, founded by former policeman Le Geng, has 27 million registered users, mostly in China, at least 2 million of whom are actively looking for dates on any given day. Technology has allowed more men, including those who may be wary of going to gay venues, to meet one another and thus to find sex partners. But it has simultaneously made it harder to reach those men with the sort of face-to-face interaction that created a sense of shared responsibility in the early years of the community response to HIV in Western countries.

The second, perhaps bigger, change is the advent of effective treatment for HIV. When AIDS invaded the gay bars of San Francisco, Sydney, London and Amsterdam, it was a visible and terrible syndrome that led to a rapid and often painful death. By the time Beijing, Shanghai, Qingdao and Chengdu had active gay scenes, AIDS was practically a thing of the past. HIV, of course, is very much alive, and spreading rapidly. But most gay men in China have probably never seen a person with symptomatic AIDS. The fear factor that comes from seeing your friends and loved-ones die is simply no longer there. This is of course a very good thing. But it does mean that it is harder to convince people of the need to take measures to protect themselves from the virus.This new reality has not been well understood by Chinese health authorities; they continue to speak of the importance of "awareness", as though gay men would change their behaviour if only they were more aware of HIV and knew how to prevent it. But new cases of HIV infection are on the rise in gay communities worldwide, even in countries where prevention knowledge is

100%. Although the Chinese language makes no distinction between HIV and AIDS in daily speech, the fact is that the two are not synonymous. Treatment has broken the inevitable progression from invisible HIV infection to visible illness (symptomatic AIDS) to death. Treatable HIV infection simply doesn't elicit the same kind of community response as AIDS once did, and no amount of "awareness-raising" will change that.

"Health concerns, including HIV, should be very important to the gay community," said Lingping Cai, who runs the China HIV/AIDS Information Network (CHAIN), a non-governmental organisation supporting HIV prevention and care efforts. "But it's hard to convince people of that. There are natural leaders in the gay community but they think about being able to come out, about equal rights in employment, about gay marriage. These are the important issues for them now – things like making internet platforms for gay friendly jobs. They are not really working on health."

Following the strategies that worked with other risk populations, HIV officials in government have tried to address the HIV epidemic in gay men by starting small pilot studies offering biomedical solutions, including circumcision and pre-exposure prophylaxis or PREP, in which HIV-negative people take antiretroviral drugs every day to help them stay uninfected. The PREP study was a typically bold experiment on China's part; though very effective as a prevention method, it has proven politically controversial in many countries. For example, in early 2016, the politically conservative government in the UK was still not providing PREP to gay men at risk for HIV, despite a good evidence base and very strong demand from the gay community. In China, the opposite problem arose: though the government offered PREP, gay men were not willing to take it – perhaps a throwback to the days when the quality of antiretroviral drugs in China was poor and side-effects common. In a feasibility study in three eastern provinces, only 197 out of 1,033 uninfected gay men surveyed said they would be willing to take the medicine to protect themselves from HIV and only 26 men – just 2.5% of the study population – actually took it. A rather higher proportion of men said they would be willing to be circumcised to prevent catching HIV, but only 3% actually showed up for their appointments and underwent the procedure.

Other than awareness raising, the main approach to preventing HIV among gay men in China is currently to test as many of them as possible for HIV and to put those who test positive on antiretroviral drugs, both for their own benefit and to reduce the likelihood that they might pass HIV on to others. According to CHAIN's Lingping Cai, the approach doesn't match the needs and desires of gay men. "Because of community movements, gay people are expressing themselves more and there's more [social] acceptance. What gay men demand is respect. But the response strategy is still medical. The strategy is to test, the intervention is to draw blood, and the output is a testing target achieved. There's no respect for human beings." Faced with this new challenge, she said, it was more necessary than ever to design prevention programmes around the needs and desires of communities. "We need a strategy for humans, not for a disease."

Again, the government is aware that strategies that worked with sex workers, drug users and people so poor they sold blood for money – socially marginalised communities sometimes living on the wrong side of the law – will not necessarily work for young, educated men scattered throughout all the major cities of the nation. Health authorities are casting around for solutions. "I've even heard a senior government official wonder aloud if legalising gay marriage might reduce risk among gay men," said Le Geng. "He was speaking personally. But still, the government is growing more and more pragmatic in the face of all these new infections. They have no other choice."

Certainly, the government agrees that community groups should be involved in the response, and it has taken steps to support such groups. To understand the current position, we need to look at how the funding streams for HIV in China have changed in the decade since the government pledged to tackle the epidemic head-on.

Taking over the purse strings

As we have seen, almost all of the early response to HIV in China was foreign-funded. From the start of the epidemic to 2009, China received over US$526 million from some 40 foreign agencies and foundations. The money was spent on 276 separate projects; though all were implemented in partnership with Chinese authorities, many were driven by the priorities and interests of the international partners. Even after China began firmly to set its own national priorities with the "Four Frees and One Care" commitment of 2004, funding for implementation was often provided by foreign sources. The first large-scale treatment services for people infected while selling plasma were mainly paid for by the Global Fund, for example. But as those services rolled out in provinces most affected by poor plasma collection practices, the government realised that it could not neglect other populations. It began to fund large-scale testing and provision of treatment to other populations out of the national budget. Details of China's spending on HIV are shown in Figure 8 of the Appendix. From an initial contribution of CNY100 million in 2001, spending increased astronomically to reach CNY3.7 billion by 2015. As the proportion of HIV-related funding coming out of national pockets grew, so did the government's desire to reduce the fragmentation that comes of having so many different foreign partners funding so many different projects.

The international community had themselves recognised this problem as early as 2003 and had tried to address it by agreeing on three rules to try to bring all elements in a country's response into a single coherent framework. Known as the "Three Ones", the rules were: one agreed national HIV/AIDS Action Framework within which all partners work; one National AIDS Coordinating Authority, and one agreed country level Monitoring and Evaluation System.

Though badly needed by countries that were being pulled in different directions by different donors, these rules were roundly ignored by the very organisations that dreamed them up. "China was the first country to step up and say: we don't want to run our national programme as just the sum of a lot of different projects," said Bernhard Schwartländer, who represented UNAIDS in Beijing at the time China began to take full control of its response to HIV. The Chinese government had previously developed five-year plans to guide the national response. However, they had never before taken charge of the contribution of foreign-funded projects to that response. CRIMS was a very important first step in unifying the response – it was certainly the first example of the sort of unified, government-led national monitoring and evaluation system envisaged by the Three Ones. Another radical step was taken in 2010, when the government rolled four separate Global Fund-backed programmes, each managed by a different entity, into a Rolling Continuation Channel which put all of the programmes firmly under national leadership.

The government did more than just assume ownership of money from foreign sources; it significantly increased the amount it spent on HIV from domestic coffers. The proportion continued to rise until, by 2014, over 99% of funds for HIV programmes in China came from domestic sources. "The leap in commitment as China took charge of its epidemic was astonishing," said Schwartländer. "It was an amazing time." Other important policy changes were also made at this time, including the end of the ban on HIV-infected foreigners visiting China.

An additional spur to national ownership of the response came from a commentary published in the influential US-based journal *Foreign Policy* by the former US government and WHO health policy adviser Jack Chow. In the July 2010 issue of *Foreign Policy*, Chow launched a blistering attack on China for taking a billion dollars from the Global Fund, a multilateral mechanism that was intended to help the world's poorest countries cope with HIV, TB and malaria.

> *It is audacious for China to assert that it needs international health assistance on par with the world's poorest countries. In fact, at the same time it is drawing from the Global Fund, China is building its entire global image as one of economic growth, accumulating wealth and international stature. To boost its public profile and prestige, China spent billions to host the Beijing Olympics and the Shanghai World Expo. Surely it could spend another $1 billion of its cash on health as well.[57]*

Though China is also a contributor to the Global Fund, it was taking out far more than it put in. Chow argued that poor countries were unable to get funding because China's successful bids were using up so many of the available resources. But, he said, neither the poor countries that were losing out nor the rich countries that were underwriting the fund dared to complain, for fear of damaging relations with China, an increasingly important investment partner for rich and poor nations alike.

The article prompted a rapid rethink at the Global Fund's headquarters in Geneva. From November 2011, China and a number of other middle-income countries were "graduated" from the Fund – they would no longer be eligible to apply for grants. On the Chinese side, "It was a slap in the face," according to one government official. "After SARS the government had really taken on board that it was responsible for the health of its citizens. That article made everyone so ashamed." The government did not even apply for the transition funds that would have helped smooth the passage to a post-Global Fund financing model. Funding from the Bill and Melinda Gates Foundation, which had supported access to prevention and treatment services among gay men and other groups, ended at roughly the same time.

The rapid withdrawal of foreign funds provoked headaches, especially in provinces with relatively high HIV prevalence. "We faced a very difficult situation when vast international cooperative projects pulled out of Yunnan," said Lu Lin, Director of Yunnan CDC. The provincial government faced an unexpected shortfall of CNY10 million (around US$1.6 million at the time). But Chow had been right that China's booming economy had reduced the need for the country to rely on international grants. No longer able to rely on the Global Fund or other outsiders for help, Yunnan dug into its own coffers and made up the shortfall in HIV spending itself.

Finding new platforms

As it turned out, the biggest effect of the loss of Global Fund money was not financial. It was the erosion of the voice of community groups in the response to HIV.

Since the earliest World Bank-funded projects of the early 2000s, foreign funders had encouraged the Chinese government to engage with civil society on the issue of HIV. But it was the Global Fund that formalised their participation in planning and delivering HIV prevention and care services. In every country, Global Fund proposals and grants are governed by a Country Coordinating Mechanism or CCM, which must include representatives from government, international partners, and civil society organisations. No civil society representation, no cash; it's that simple. What's more, in China the Global Fund stipulated as a condition of providing a grant that a certain proportion of the funding should go to NGOs: a fifth for the first and second round of grants, half for the third and all of the money for the fourth.

As was seen in Chapter 3, there was no body of established NGOs in China, so this presented something of a challenge. Many groups sprang up to absorb the money – around 1,000 by 2012. The process was not always an easy one. There were no clear mechanisms in Chinese law through which these community organisations could even establish themselves as legal entities. Springing up from nothing, they naturally lacked organisational capacity, and some of them were also somewhat opportunistic. "Some of the NGOs see the community as a client, as a source of money, nothing more. But communities are not stupid: they know when an NGO is doing nothing for their rights," said CHAIN's Lingping Cai.

In addition, many Chinese officials resented the imposition of these groups. In the past, they had used government channels to reach those most likely to be in need of HIV services – former plasma sellers, drug users and sex workers. "But the gay community is different [from plasma sellers, drug users or sex workers]; it's more diffuse," explained Ray Yip, who directed both the US CDC and the Bill and Melinda Gates Foundation AIDS programmes in China. The need to adopt new approaches to reach gay men combined with the need to meet the stringent rules of the Global Fund led to a change in attitudes among officials in the central government."In China, international supporters pushed gay-men-based NGOs to become part of the response. That has forced CDCs and NGOs to work together, which is not an easy alliance," Yip said. "But over the years it has created higher level political permission for this arrangement. There's still quite a bit of animosity and discomfort on both sides, but at the top political level, they see NGOs as necessary but not sufficient, and CDCs and the medical establishment as necessary but not sufficient. So now, both sides respect this compromise as a necessary part of the solution."

Community-based organisations say that they learned a great deal from their interaction with the Global Fund, and through that with government authorities. "There were a few community organisations before the Global Fund, but they were mostly just doing peer outreach. With the support of the Fund, we moved into operations research, advocacy, anti-stigma work, all kinds of things," said Lin Meng, of CAP+, who represented civil society organisations on the Country Coordinating Mechanism, the Global Fund's governing body in China. "Participating in the CCM also helped us to understand how democracy operates, what the rules and procedures should be. This was important knowledge for civil society; we learned about rights, respect, all sorts of things. During the process I had to deal with governments, donors, international organisations, academics in institutes. I learned how to work with them and how to fight for something, how to negotiate. The impact of the Fund was huge."

After the Global Fund announced that it would no longer be supporting programmes in China, there was a great deal of concern about the fate of these non-governmental organisations. In some areas of the country, for example in Yunnan, local authorities recognised the vital contribution they could make in working with marginalised populations. "We need to cling vigorously to grass-roots institutions and move the key battleground to the communities and rural areas," said Lin Lu, director of Yunnan province's CDC. "It makes AIDS prevention and control more tangible and specific." However as we saw earlier, the closure of major foreign-funded programmes left the province with large hole in its budget. The Yunnan government itself created a fund which mirrored the procedures of the Global Fund. "The bidding procedure is organised by NGOs and assessed by experts from several fields," said Lin Lu. His colleague Xiping Huan, head of the AIDS Division in Jiangsu CDC, spoke very specifically of the special role that community organisations have to play in the response, especially as the epidemic shifts to gay men as a result of social change. "From the viewpoint of the government, or society, or personally, it's very easy to just see the disease," she said. "But you have to look at what is behind the disease. I've said to community based organisations, 'You must start addressing the cultural drivers of the disease.'"

Not all local governments were as quick to recognise the potential contribution of domestic non-government partners. In May 2011, six months before China was "graduated" from the fund, the Global Fund management had frozen payments to Beijing because many provinces and prefectures were not doing enough to involve civil society.[58] NGOs and others worried that without the leverage of the Global Fund, they would have even less room to do their work. "The truth is, we failed to professionalise the NGO community, and they still find it difficult to make their voice heard," said Bernhard Schwartländer, who has served as both UNAIDS and WHO representative in China. "The CCM gave them an internal lever which has now gone."

Community groups felt the loss keenly. "If I had to describe in a word how I felt when the Global Fund pulled out, I would say 'grief'. It seems like when they left, NGOs and CBOs [community-based organisations] slipped back into silence," said CAP+'s Lin Meng. The pull-out was sudden, and there was little time to prepare alternative mechanisms for civil society participation. "It felt like we were abandoned."

The central government, however, was increasingly aware of the importance of community groups in reaching those most at risk. In December 2012, the then Vice Premier Li Keqiang met with the heads of eight NGOs involved in the HIV response. Ray Yip recalled the meeting: "He congratulated them on what they were doing, and they were very quick to point out that they were all supported by international funding, which was near the very end. What to do? And Li Keqiang said, 'Well of course we'll take over [the funding],' " the former manager of the Bill and Melinda Gates Foundation programmes in China laughed. "That was one of sweetest moments. In other countries you don't know if it will really happen, but in China, if someone at that level says that, you know it's as good as the law."

Li Keqiang was as good as his word. Because of his long-standing commitment to helping prevent HIV and care for those affected, the Premier worked tirelessly to change both the thinking and the entrenched practice of colleagues in the bureaucracy, and to set up structures that would for the first time channel government money to NGOs. By 2015 China's Ministry of Finance was providing some CNY30 million (US$5 million) for community-based organisations responding to HIV. Not content with that level of commitment, Li Keqiang topped up the funding for NGOs with another CNY20 million (US$3.2 million) from the Premier's Fund, a discretionary spending pool used mostly for natural disasters. On top of that, some provinces make extra money available to support the work of community groups.

This provision of funds to non-government groups represents a remarkable departure from regular government practice in China. Not surprisingly, there are still issues to be resolved before it functions as smoothly as everyone would like. Thomas Cai runs one of the longest-standing non-government organisations supporting people living with HIV in China. Initially, he funded all of his work himself, sometimes collecting donations from friends as well. Even then, however, it was difficult to operate. "Our group was not considered a legal entity. Overseas you call it a charity but here in China there was no legal precedent." This made it impossible to open bank accounts or track expenses, and thus difficult to prove to outside donors that money is well spent. More recently, it has become possible to register non-government groups in a single administrative area but, as CHAIN's Lingping Cai explains, it's not easy. "We need to renew our registration every year. It's expensive in terms of time and energy; it takes our finance and admin people two months every year." Many community-based groups don't make it through the registration process; they essentially become sub-contractors delivering services for CDC offices.

Since national and local CDCs and other government agencies hold the purse strings, they are able to determine what activities are undertaken by the community groups they support. In early 2016, the vast majority of that activity centred on providing testing to at-risk communities. In 2015, none of the central government money was made available to community groups wanting to do advocacy, or hoping to work to protect the rights of people with HIV, including by attacking stigma and discrimination. "We want to see NGOs being more proactive in advocacy, working to promote the rights of the groups they represent," said Lingping Cai. "But they can't because they are taking money from CDC for service delivery. It stops up their mouths."

The WHO's Bernhard Schwartländer believes these observations are legitimate. "The way NGOs are set up, well, there's no real framework for community accountability," he said. "It requires a level of trust that doesn't exist right now." However, he's optimistic that that can change. "There's an incredible seriousness of purpose among China's leaders right now; they have shown themselves to be remarkably willing to adapt," he said. "The epidemic is changing. If the government can begin to see the gay community as a source of opportunity rather than just a source of risk, then it could continue in its great progress against HIV."

Some mechanisms developed in the heady years when China's government took full charge of the national response have survived and function well. The Red Ribbon Forum, for example, is a platform that brings officials from health, public security, education and other sectors together with people from the private sector and communities to discuss sensitive issues around HIV. "Those difficult discussions used to be convened by international organisations like UNAIDS," said Catherine Sozi, who currently represents the United Nations HIV programme in China. "But Red Ribbon is a Chinese forum, with a channel to the State Council and other policy bodies. That makes it very powerful." The forum has recently brought together people to discuss the sex trade, continuing discrimination in healthcare, the challenges of hepatitis co-infection and other thorny issues. If policy-makers can learn to take these discussions seriously, regarding all participants as equal partners and integrating the contributions into plans for joint action, the country will be well placed to meet the challenges posed by the evolving HIV epidemic.

Chapter 8

HIV-Related Stigma and Discrimination in China: A Persistent Puzzle

Anuradha Chaddah and Zunyou Wu

"Should I kill my son? If I kill him, will this save my family?"

—Farmer, Anhui province, 1996

In 1996,epidemiologist Zunyou Wu, working out of the Fuyang CDC office in Anhui province, was investigating the emerging HIV epidemic that was sweeping through families that had sold plasma in central China. His work with HIV-positive populations had prepared him to answer questions regarding the disease's symptoms and prognosis, to tackle the hard reality of limited medical relief and to empathise with patients who were discovering that their lives were going to be disrupted by a disease of which they knew very little. He was not, however, prepared for the question presented to him by the agitated and visibly troubled 48-year-old-farmer who now sat across from him looking desperate and hopeless. The man had travelled for many hours by train to Fuyang to seek information, unbeknown to anyone in his family. The farmer explained that his 20-year-old-son, who was back at home in the village, was a former commercial plasma donor who had recently tested positive for HIV. The young CDC doctor nodded his head with understanding and was ready to dispense professional advice; he anticipated questions regarding possible medical therapies and the accompanying cost, as well as concerns about how to keep the man's son healthy so he could work and continue to contribute to the family's income. What he did not anticipate was the question that the distressed farmer put to him next: "Should I kill my son? If I kill him, will this save my family?"

The "Stigma Factor"

AIDS-related stigma arose even before the HIV virus was identified; it has been a major barrier to the resolution of the HIV epidemic ever since. Writing in a newspaper commentary in 2008, United Nations Secretary-General Ban Ki-moon recognised the significance of the "stigma factor". Ki-moon noted that: "One of the biggest hurdles for our global response to AIDS is psychological," and that "Almost everywhere in the world, discrimination remains a fact of daily life for people living with HIV."[59]

Those sentiments were echoed more recently by China's current President, Xi Jinping. One of Xi Jinping's earlier visits after being elected Communist Party Secretary in November 2012 was to a group of people living with HIV/AIDS in Beijing. He urged society to abandon discrimination. "HIV/AIDS is not terrible in itself, but what is really dreadful is the ignorance about HIV/AIDS and the prejudice against AIDS patients," said Xi. "Everyone living with HIV and AIDS is our brother and sister. The whole society should light their life with love."

Stigma is defined as "a mark of shame or disgrace" by Merriam-Webster Dictionary or "a strong lack of respect for a person or group of people... because they have done something society does not approve of," in Cambridge Dictionaries Online. When HIV first emerged onto the global scene in the 1980s, people were quick to characterise the disease as a "gay" disease and/or a disease of the immoral and irresponsible. These beliefs, driven in part by fear and in larger part by ignorance, moved to quickly disassociate those with the disease from mainstream society. Stigma can be experienced in several ways. An individual may perceive stigma in that they are aware that they are part of a societal stereotype; people living with HIV are aware that some portion of society assumes that they are injection drug users, sexually promiscuous or involved in immoral behaviour. Internalised stigma or self-stigma occurs when an individual accepts society's negative view of them and subsequently has a poorer self-perception or self-esteem. Shameful, disgraceful and guilty are often words used by HIV patients to describe how they feel about their disease.

When people and societies act on their feelings of disapproval or disgust, stigma is turned in to active discrimination. HIV-related discrimination is widespread and takes on many different forms in terms of housing, employment or education. All of these forms of discrimination, and more, are routinely experienced by those living with HIV. Given the myriad ways in which HIV-related stigma is experienced by the average person diagnosed with the disease, it is not surprising that HIV-related stigma affects all aspects of HIV care from implementation of disease prevention behaviours, test-seeking, care-seeking and the quality of care provided to those who test positive.

Sowing fear, reaping stigma

While HIV prevalence in China remains relatively low at less than 0.1% nationally, HIV stigma is widespread. In China, HIV is widely considered to be a disease of the marginalised; people who inject drugs or who sell or buy sex. The disease is also associated with men who have sex with men, another group considered to be on the fringe of mainstream society. Until 2001, homosexuality was officially considered to be a mental illness in China.[60] Traditionally, Chinese culture embraces concepts of familial harmony and "getting along" over that of individuality and "making waves." In this conformist social context, those who are regarded as behaving outside of the norm are judged harshly and seen as deserving of whatever hardship befalls them. Stigma and discrimination flow inevitably from such judgements.

The 2009 China Stigma Index survey, which was one of the first such surveys conducted in the world, aimed to document and "quantify" HIV-related stigma in China by analysing the experience of over 2,000 people living with HIV. Being HIV-positive overwhelmingly led to feelings of shame (62%) and low self-esteem (75%). Over half of the women and over 40% of the men surveyed had contemplated suicide since finding out about their infection.[61]

China's early response to HIV, as described in Chapter 1, did little to minimise this stigmatisation and laid the groundwork for much of the discrimination that is experienced by those who live with HIV in China today. When the first cases of HIV were diagnosed in China in the late 1980s, the disease was immediately characterised as a "capitalist" disease of the rich and hedonistic West. This quickly led to those Chinese with the disease being labelled as "foreign" or outside of Chinese society.

Early public health warnings regarding the risks of HIV were often accompanied by stark and frightening images of gaunt and disease-ridden Africans; not only did these images underline the "foreign" nature of the illness, but they also led to HIV disease quickly being associated in people's minds as a terrifying, automatic death sentence. The cover of one book dedicated to the global HIV epidemic, published by the Heilongjiang People's Press in 1987, showed a bleeding heart pierced by a skull-topped arrow with the word "AIDS" looming over the image. Such fear-mongering laid a strong foundation for the inevitable lash of discrimination that was to fall upon those who contracted HIV in China.

To make matters worse, HIV wasn't just associated with foreigners in China, but with a particular type of foreigner – gay men – a population that was already frowned upon at home. Then, when indigenous infections did begin to surface, they appeared in another group seen as degenerate outsiders: drug injectors from poor families in rural areas, many of them members of ethnic minorities.

To this day, the extent of HIV-related stigma and discrimination in China is described by people living with the disease as being widespread and touching every aspect of their daily lives, even 30 years after the disease first appeared in the country. Research data affirm these assertions. In a 2009 survey of 3,968 Chinese adults from a combination of cities, town and rural areas, 72% said that an HIV-positive co-worker should not be allowed to continue to work; 58% said that if a family member became ill with the disease they would want that fact to remain a secret, and 34% of them would not be willing to take care of that family member or allow them to remain in their household. In the same year, a Kaiser Family Foundation survey found that close to a quarter of Americans would not be prepared to work with someone with HIV (and another 29% would feel uncomfortable doing so). Only one in four Americans said they would be prepared to share a house with an infected housemate, though the question did not, as in China, refer specifically to a family member.[62]

Understanding that HIV-related stigma and discrimination are serious impediments to the effective treatment of the HIV epidemics in China, health officials are eager to combat such attitudes, but are not necessarily aware of how to accomplish their goals. While education, public awareness, healthcare policies and robust legal protections have worked around the globe to combat HIV stigma, until the late 20th century China's approach to the problem had been paradoxical at best, and largely ineffective.

Supportive families are not the norm

In Chinese culture, the centrality of one's family to ones identity and security is paramount. Familial bonds are considered sacrosanct, transcending those created by one's business, school and friendships. On the surface, this might seem promising for people living with HIV: one would hopefully be able to rely on the support of their nearest and dearest. In practice, however, the importance of honouring one's family and strong self-stigmatisation, which leads to feelings of shame and disgrace, often prevents people with HIV from seeking familial support. A 2009 survey of people living with HIV in China found that 40% were not able to tell their parents of their diagnosis, for fear of being rejected outright by the family unit. Stories such as the one at the beginning of this chapter highlight the blame that families often place upon an HIV-positive family member and the concern that allowing the individual to remain part of the family will be catastrophic for the unit's survival. When a family member is revealed to be HIV-positive, often other family will automatically assume that individuals have behaved in some "immoral" way. In addition, although HIV is actually a rather fragile virus which is impossible to contract through casual contact, the fear-mongering of the early years has left many people in China with a greatly exaggerated sense of its transmissibility. Endless awareness campaigns do not seem to have been able to dent the belief that HIV is highly infectious. In 2002, an HIV-related NGO worker told Human Rights Watch that if you were known to be HIV-positive: "Your family won't eat with you, they give you food to eat apart from them, and they won't have contact with you. Your friends ignore you... If you pass them a cigarette, the won't accept it."[63]

Though perhaps less universal over a decade later, these behaviours persist in China. As recently as 2014, an NCAIDS survey of people living with HIV found that a fifth had been allocated dedicated tableware by their family; a slightly higher proportion reported that their clothes were washed separately from those of their family members.[64]

Families themselves fear that they will be stigmatised and face discrimination if they do not reject an HIV-positive family member. Stories from rural China of entire families being shunned because one family member tests HIV-positive are numerous; villagers have refused to buy vegetables from such families, or to sell their own produce to them. The family members of people with HIV get turned away from the village bathhouse for fear that they will spread the virus. Though these stories were more common a decade ago, they continue to surface now.

In this context, many HIV-positive people in China still don't share their diagnosis with their family or friends; the secrecy is a way of protecting their loved ones. As one HIV-positive Chinese man explained in 2015: "I am more afraid of the stigma than the illness itself because nothing can hurt me more than people looking down on my parents."[65]

Being stripped of familial support leaves those who are HIV-positive even more vulnerable to isolation, shame and guilt. Kerong Wang, Deputy Head Nurse at Beijing's Ditan Hospital, cared extensively for AIDS patients during the 1990s and recalls the abandonment her patients often had to endure. "In the 1990s, people had a very limited understanding of AIDS," she said. "The mere mentioning of the word AIDS was frightening enough. Our patient ward once had a businesswoman. She seemed quite rich. From what she told us, she had many, many friends. Then she was found with AIDS and became a patient at our hospital. Every day she'd look out of the window in great hope. Two months passed, however, and no one came to visit her. Her daily supplies were all purchased by us nurses."

Wang remembered the gratitude that this patient showed for even the smallest acts of kindness. "One time she was craving for tomatoes. After my shift I went to the market and bought her two big and juicy tomatoes. She took out 200 kuai [Yuan] from her purse and said to me, crying, It's almost Children's Day. Get your kid a nice gift..." The patient died shortly thereafter, Wang said. "While going over her personal belongings I found a letter in the form of a will. In the letter she thanked us for taking care of her and offered to donate her body to medical research. Her decision was very moving. Her story showed us all the more clearly how lonely AIDS patients could feel deep down and all the more why they especially need the caring and understanding of their family, friends and society in general."

Losing the support of one's family places an emotional burden on an HIV-positive individual, but it can also leave them in difficulty when it comes to life's basics such as food and housing. One person who has tried to fill the gap is Thomas Cai, who set up AIDS Care China, one of the first organisations providing support for people with HIV in the country. He recalled how hard it was at first to help people who had been diagnosed with HIV in China's cities. "Most of the [HIV] patients were drug users... When they left the hospital, they went back to the streets or were living under bridges," Cai said. He tried to provide housing for these men and women, renting several flats, but found that the residents were constantly forced out. "The first guy was forced to move three times during three months because of neighbours, they cut the supply of water and electricity, and even called the police," Cai remembered. "I was really confused. We raise pets, keep plants, but we can't accept a real person, we can't give them room to live. During that time, I felt both fulfilment and pain."

"Innocence" is no protection

Most accounts of the roots of HIV-related stigma, like this one, point to the early association of virus with extramarital sex and drug use – behaviours that many in society enjoy, but most at least pretend to disapprove of. In China, one might expect things to be different, because of the events described in Chapter 2. Tens of thousands of Chinese citizens, perhaps hundreds of thousands, were infected with HIV while selling their blood. Even those who believed that HIV was somehow a punishment for taking drugs or having extramarital sex could not extend that logic to those infected during plasma collection. And yet the massive epidemic of the mid-

1990s does not seem to have in any way diminished the stigma associated with HIV in China.

Discrimination is even visited on children who have only the most peripheral association with the virus. Close to one in ten people living with HIV in China surveyed in 2009 reported that their children had been kicked out of school. And again, these cases continue, long after the government has committed to care for individuals and families in need. In 2011 the *Peninsula Morning Post* reported on the story of Xiao Ai (Little Ai), a 14-year-old, HIV-positive boy from Dandon Kuandian Manchu Autonomous County who attended an "exclusive" school for one. Xiao Ai was born with HIV. Both of his parents were infected with the virus but did not become aware of their HIV-positive status until shortly prior to their son's birth. When Xiao Ai was seven years old and clamouring to start school, other parents in the village petitioned the school to exclude him from being in class with their children. The school conceded, and eventually the village decided to build a school that only Xiao Ai attends, outside of the village. At the time of the story's publication, Xiao Ai had been attending school for seven years and never hada single classmate.[66]

More recently an even more startling story involving an HIV-positive child was reported by Shenzhen satellite TV. On 7 December 2014, 203 villagers from Shufangya village in the south-western province of Sichuan convened a special meeting to discuss whether eight-year-old Kunkun, a boy who had lived his entire life in this village with this grandfather, should be allowed to continue to live there. Kunkun had recently been discovered to be HIV-positive when he had received treatment at a local hospital for an unrelated bump to the head. With the child and his grandfather present at the meeting, the villagers shared their concerns regarding Kunkun's continued residence in the village; one villager noted: "If he [has] an injury [with] bleeding, he will be infectious. So, if he is not isolated, the infectivity for future generations is very serious." After less than thirty minutes of discussion, the villagers voted to expel Kunkun and his grandfather from the village.[67]

Children with HIV/AIDS and the uninfected offspring of those with the disease are particularly vulnerable victims of the epidemic. These children are either sick themselves, left to take care of ailing parents, orphaned, or a combination thereof. They have no means for providing for their basic survival needs such as food, clothing and shelter. Furthermore, they are rarely in a position to secure necessary medical resources.

Legislative challenges and conflicts

Under China's Employment Promotion Law, "Employers should not deny employment for the reason that the applicant carries pathogens of infectious disease." More specifically to HIV/AIDS, the Regulation on the Prevention and Control of AIDS, which was issued by the State Council in 2006, clearly states: "Employers and individuals should not discriminate against people living with HIV, AIDS patients, or their family members...The rights and interests of people living with HIV/AIDS, patients and their family members concerning their marriages, employment, healthcare, and education are protected by law."

But sometimes HIV-positive employees were effectively unprotected from having the widespread stigma and discrimination that they face in their personal seep into their work lives.

Lin Meng, who was diagnosed with HIV two decades ago and who founded the China Alliance of People Living with HIV/AIDS in 2004, poignantly expresses the deep frustration and pain felt on the part of the HIV-positivepopulation who are left unshielde "We [have] such a long narrative linking the disease with bad people, such a long labelling and moralising" Meng said these lower-level regulations are in clear violation of the laws passed by the National People's Congress. "The laws like the labour laws do protect the rights of people with HIV, this is very clear, they look very beautiful. But at the implementation level there are lots of ministerial regulations and policies that contradict the beautiful laws, and those are the ones people choose to implement."

Discrimination in the workplace isn't just about being allowed to work, Meng noted, it's also about being treated with dignity. He described his own experience working in the offices of the National Institute of Public Health Education, where his

AIDS support organisation was based. "One day I went to the canteen for lunch and a group of leaders of the institute were there and they stopped me from going to the public canteen. They were almost apologetic saying,'It's true, we are a public health institute, but still many people don't understand, so it would be better for you not to go the canteen.' I felt angry, ashamed, but I couldn't express it." Meng is a quiet, largely cheerful man, but he was visibly upset by the memory. "That was 2004. Other colleagues then invited me to go out to a restaurant, ordered lots of dishes; they felt terrible and wanted to support me. They felt so bad that the environment wasn't more supportive." Despite support from these individuals, the environment at the workplace was poisoned. "Overnight my relationship with my colleagues crashed," said Meng.

Over a decade later, state institutions are increasingly aware of laws that prohibit HIV-related discrimination in the workplace and some, at least, appear reluctant to violate those laws outright. This has not, however, greatly improved the welfare of those the law seeks to protect, as the story of Mao Mao (not his real name) illustrates. Mao had been a middle school teacher for over a decade in Zhejiang Province and was stopped from teaching when he was diagnosed as HIV positive. "They continued to pay my salary, but said I couldn't teach anymore," Mao recounted. He was devastated: he loved his job, and could think of nothing that would justify this sudden decision.

Concerned about HIV-related discrimination in the workplace in China, NCAIDS collaborated with the International Labour Organization in 2010 to summarise what was known. They reported a survey of 1,000 Chinese employees by researchers at the Chinese University of Political Science and Law which found that one in two workers believed that HIV-positive employees should be "deprived of equal employment". Of the 200 respondents who were business managers with the authority to hire workers, two-thirds believed that HIV-positive workers should not have equal employment opportunities. Some of these same managers admitted to using employment ads that clearly stated, "Potential employees should be clear of infectious diseases such as HIV and AIDS." A 2007 survey published by the *Chinese Journal of Clinical Psychology* found that nine out of every ten respondents reported having lost at least one job after testing positive for HIV. Such behaviour by employers, while undisputedly bigoted, needs to be placed in context. The NCAIDS report also details a survey of employees published by the *Chinese Health and Education* journal that found that 81% of respondents would not buy any product made by people with HIV.[68] Knowing this, employers might well see HIV-positive employees as a financial liability for their business.

Given the legal quagmire described above, it is not surprising that few HIV-positive employees seek legal redress for the employment woes. Just as breaches of confidentiality laws by the healthcare systems go unpunished, so go violations of the anti-discrimination labour laws. Additionally, employees are disincentivised to come forward with their complaints because they don't want their disease status to be even more widely exposed to the broader public and to other potential future employers. Wronged employees are more likely to avoid litigation and cling to anonymity in the hopes of quickly moving onto the next job.

There are, however, encouraging signs that things are beginning to change. In 2013, a plaintiff for the first time won an HIV-related employment discrimination case in China. A teacher from Jianxi, Ms. Qi, saw her application for a teaching position rejected by a school because she was living with HIV. Qi's case was the fourth such lawsuit against schools in China, but the first that ended in victory for a teacher. Qi was awarded CNY45,000 (US$7,200) in compensation.[69]

Stigma and discrimination in the healthcare system

One of the most extraordinary paradoxes of China's response to HIV is found in its healthcare system. On the one hand, China has done more than any other country of its income level to provide free or affordable HIV treatment and care to its citizens. On the other hand, people with HIV are routinely denied surgery and other services in the country's hospitals and clinics, their privacy is rarely respected, and healthcare professionals frequently treat them without the compassion or dignity they deserve.

There are, of course, exceptions. Nurse Wang, who described her experience caring for people abandoned by family and friends earlier in this chapter, was one of them. Her dedication was so out of the ordinary that she received the Nationwide Outstanding Professional Award, and was elected a representative of Beijing's Tenth National Congress of the Communist Party. To this day, many health staff still treat people with HIV with less compassion than other patients. Healthcare providers discriminate against HIV-positive patients in several ways, including: by directly refusing to treat a patient or by unnecessarily referring the patient to another healthcare facility, by delivering inappropriate or substandard care or by providing care without the requisite respect for the patient's rights, such as the patient's right to confidentiality.

In 2012, the story of Xiaofeng, a 25-year-old HIV-positive man from Tianjin, turned the spotlight on discrimination in China's healthcare system. Having been diagnosed with lung cancer and advised to have surgery, Xiaofeng sought surgical treatment at two different hospitals. The medical professionals acknowledged that Xiaofeng needed the surgery in order to survive, but he was denied treatment once physicians at each establishment found out he was HIV-positive. Desperate to receive the care he needed, Xiaofeng approached a third medical institution and concealed his HIV-positive status from the medical staff. Only then was he operated upon.

China's laws prohibit medical facilities from refusing to treat people with HIV, and Xiaofeng sued the Cancer Institute and Hospital of Tianjin Medical University.[70] His action is a sign that a few people with HIV in China are beginning to stand up for their rights, and that the courts are beginning to take them seriously. But Xiaofeng's story is not an isolated case. The 2009 survey of HIV-positive individuals found that 14% had experienced discrimination on the part of a medical professional or medical institution. Routine HIV testing in hospital and clinic settings has increased massively since then, so the possibility for concealing one's HIV status in order to access treatment for unrelated conditions has diminished. In 2013, over 8% of HIV-positive people responding to an NCAIDS survey said they had been denied treatment because of their infection.

The irrational fear and enduring stigma associated with HIV even among healthcare workers is a challenge for China's policy-makers. One of the obstacles to scaling up HIV treatment is the difficulty of finding physicians who are willing to do the work. A 2009 study found that 33% of China's healthcare workers would request to be assigned elsewhere if faced with treating an HIV-positive patient. Part of this is bare-faced discrimination, related to the stigma associated with the virus.

The government has since set up nine dedicated training centres to teach doctors to provide HIV-related care. Many provincial health bureaus now provide salary supplements, promotions and other incentives to persuade more doctors and nurses to care for HIV-positive patients.

Enlisting help in the battle against HIV-related stigma

In common with other countries, the Chinese government has tried to enlist the help of celebrities and other high-profile people to show support for people who are affected by HIV. One of the earliest examples dates from the late 1990s, and it came about almost by accident.

Virologist Yi Zeng, one of the AIDS warriors whose work was described in Chapter 3, had been trying unsuccessfully to get well-known figures to support AIDS campaigns. Then, on a flight from Taiyuan back to Beijing, he found himself sitting next to Taiwanese-American pop idol Fei Xiang (also known by his American name, Kris Phillips). "I thought this would be a great opportunity to talk directly with a real celebrity!" recalled Zeng. "We started talking and I told him about my work with AIDS, saying that we were interested in working with people in the entertainment industry to educate the public. I asked if he would come with me to visit some patients and he immediately said yes. I said we would buy some flowers and fruit for him to give the patients, then go to visit the patients together, but he said no, that he was the one visiting them and he would buy the flowers."

Knowing that the tall, good-looking pop star would cut quite a figure in Beijing's Ditan Hospital, the virologist let TV reporters know of the visit. "Kris came with a couple of dozen bouquets of flowers, walking right into the hospital rooms with them. After he met with the patients and gave them the flowers, he said that he had to hug them like he was used to in the United States. He hugged every single patient." Zeng particularly remembered the reaction of one of the patients who was most seriously ill. "As soon as he came into the hospital room, Kris walked up to him and gave him a hug and asked how he was; the young man immediately started crying." The visit was broadcast on TV. "It received a lot of attention," Zeng recalled.

At first, it was not easy to get others to follow the pop star's example. According to one person who has worked to raise the profile of HIV in China, celebrities were at first keener to put their names to campaigns to protect the environment or reduce poverty. Xinlun Wang, an AIDS education specialist who works with a group that coordinates celebrities to participate in AIDS awareness campaigns, recalled the early years: "In 2000, AIDS was still a very sensitive topic for the general public. It was extremely difficult to sign up AIDS Ambassadors. We couldn't find them, we didn't know of their interest for public welfare, and mostly, we did not know celebrities who would consent to have their image connected with AIDS."

"We started to search for celebrities blindly, and desperately, like headless chickens". Thankless efforts and constant disappointment left Wang's group deflated, but one day in August 2000 they were surprised by the answer of one of the most famous actors of the time, Cunxi Pu, who agreed to join the cause.He emphatically commented, "Not a problem! It is my honour and duty to work in HIV/AIDS prevention, and be an advocate. I hope I inspire others to join in as well!" Later that year, the Ministry of Health held a press conference announcing Pu as their very first AIDS Ambassador. In appointing Pu, Vice Minister of Health Dakui Yin, declared: "You are the team leader for the AIDS education programme, and I am on your team!" That team of AIDS advocates has since expanded to include singers, actors and well-known sports stars. In 2004,for example, the National Basketball Association aired a series of TV spots in the U.S. and China showing Yao Ming, a beloved Chinese national who played for the Houston Rockets, playing basketball, embracing and eating a meal with NBA superstar Magic Johnson, who was widely known to be HIV-positive.

China's political leaders have also been actively involved in positively reshaping the nation's view of those living with HIV. In 2003, Chinese media carried stories featuring Premier Wen Jiabao shaking hands with HIV-positive plasma donors. This was the first time a top leader from the Chinese government publicly shared their concern and care for patients with HIV. The Premier began to participate in World AIDS Day events every year – he accompanied President Hu Jintao on the visit to AIDS patients at a Beijing hospital in 2004, described in Chapter 4. Health officials expected the Premier to turn his attention to other priorities as time went by, but his commitment remained so strong that his office actively pushed the Ministry of Health to arrange HIV-related events in which he could participate. Flying with health officials to visit AIDS orphans one year, Premier Wen Jiabao said he felt compelled to keep bringing the issue to the nation's attention. 'There are 365 days in each year, I have to use at least one for AIDS,' he said. And so he did, for all 10 years of his Premiership.

Showing commitment to the destigmatisation of those living with HIV, the Premier followed up on the day before World AIDS Day in 2007 by visiting the village of Wenlou. Because of Wenlou's status as Henan province's most heavily affected AIDS village, produce grown by the village's farmers was nearly impossible to sell. The Premier recognised the way in which HIV/AIDS stigma plagued the villagers' everyday lives. "AIDS stigma is still a serious issue in our society, and people still lack sufficient scientific knowledge about it. We should have more educational campaigns to raise awareness and reduce stigma." He backed this call with a highly-visible act, remarking to a farmer: "You can tell everyone that the Premier visited Wenlou today and ate vegetables grown here."

More recently, HIV has found an important advocate in the country's First Lady, Peng Liyuan, who has made numerous television appearances with AIDS orphans and serves as a WHO goodwill ambassador for tuberculosis and HIV/AIDS. Her efforts to erode the stigma associated with HIV in China have encouraged others to follow suit.

Each year Peng Liyuan invites children affected by HIV to participate in summer camps and makes appearances during World AIDS Day to spread HIV awareness. A famous folk singer, the only song Peng Liyuan publically sings nowadays is "Fly the Red Ribbon", whose lyrics express her concern and care for children affected by AIDS. Describing what motivates her to try and improve life for these children, the First Lady said:

I've visited HIV/AIDS patients in the hospitals before, and met with families affected by AIDS, been in close contact with adults and children alike. The children and orphans that I met gave me a most lasting impression, with their innocent and hopeful eyes. For many of them, AIDS took away their parents and other loved ones. They are too young for these pressures, this family burden, this poverty, this loneliness. Their faces, stricken with anguish, have aged far too quickly. Yet when we eat together or play games, they are just like other children. They have beautiful ideas and goals, full of hope but others' misguided understandings, discrimination and cruel ostracising have created unbelievable emotional hurdles incomprehensible by an average person. They struggle with abject poverty, feelings of inferiority, and alienation, and deserve even more caring, understanding and assistance.

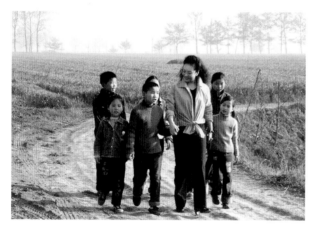

Peng Liyuan with children affected by HIV/AIDS, in field (2006)

In the last few years I have participated in many HIV/AIDS related public service activities, and through my numerous interactions with those affected I have come to learn more. To them, suffering from the disease and threat of death is less painful than the discrimination, seclusion, cold indifference and avoidance of those around them. Societal discrimination is a primary reason for HIV/AIDS-affected individuals to feel completely backed into a corner, but it's rooted in society's misinformation, and lack of education about the disease. As such, it is imperative that we engage in widespread education about HIV/AIDS, its prevention. People will more widely understand transmission that daily interactions at work and school will not lead to infection. Together we can fight stigma, and adverse reactions to the disease will slowly disappear. Only then can we truly fight AIDS together, creating a society for those affected that is harmonious.

Media reporting of anti-discrimination cases such as that won by teacher Qi combined with the efforts of politicians and celebrities may begin to put a dent in China's stubborn aversion to dealing fairly with those affected by HIV. China's healthcare workforce of over 5 million could provide the largest lever for further progress. They need to be better educated about the virus and to step up as the leading luminaries on how to care for and respect the rights of people who live with HIV, their families and communities. Accomplishing this goal will be a challenge, but given the country's significant achievements over the past 30 years, it should not be impossible.

Chapter 9

Building on the Past, Facing the Future

Zunyou Wu and Elizabeth Pisani

In the three decades since the first AIDS case was identified in China, much has been tried and learned, and a great deal has changed, as we hope this book has shown. The wall of xenophobia that first greeted the disease was undermined by the discovery of domestic transmission among drug injectors and plasma sellers, but that in turn was quickly covered by the reluctance of the government at that time to acknowledge the problem lasting through much of the second decade of the epidemic. Now, in 2016, the picture looks very different indeed. China is open about its evolving HIV epidemic, and is working actively and pragmatically to reduce the spread of the virus, including through the world's largest methadone programme for former drug injectors. The country also operates the world's largest HIV testing programme, performing some 144 million HIV tests in 2015, many of them in the groups most at risk of infection. It is this active testing programme that opened the door for another of the country's great achievements: the provision of care and antiretroviral therapy to hundreds of thousands of citizens, many of them living in rural areas. The rapid progress in providing treatment and care for those infected has been truly astonishing.

Building success over 30 years

In this short summary chapter, we try to distil the lessons of the past 30 years, and to highlight the factors which have been critical to China's success. We also outline the challenges that remain, and suggest some of the pathways for the future.

Listening, trying, measuring

One of the most important building blocks for China's success was the early experimental approach to HIV prevention in groups at high risk. With little domestic experience dealing with epidemics driven by sex or drug-taking, Chinese scientists and officials took every opportunity to learn from experience in other countries. Opening their minds to all possibilities, they read scientific papers and consulted with foreign colleagues and professionals (including professional sex workers). They travelled to observe different ways of doing things. And though they were not always comfortable with what they saw or heard, they were determined to try out proven approaches at home. Importantly, most of these early experiments fused intervention with research approaches, meaning that everything that was tried was rigorously documented. Over time, this small group of health officials and academics built up a very solid evidence base about what worked and what didn't in the Chinese situation. In the early years, there was only a limited opportunity to act on the results of these experiments. But the academics saw to it that information was carefully documented, and when possible published in credible academic publications, ready to draw on when the time was right.

"Best practice" is not always best: daring to be different

China learned a lot from international partners early in the epidemic. But local scientists and authorities were always careful to adapt what they learned to local conditions. China, with its vast population and strong, centralised government structures, is in many ways unique. China's HIV epidemic also developed in ways rarely seen in other countries. Significant outbreaks related to medical practices were recorded among orphans in Romania and in a handful of other places, but nothing like on the scale of the HIV outbreak among farmers who sold plasma in China's central provinces.

These unique characteristics arguably demanded (and also facilitated) a unique response, one which did not necessarily follow internationally accepted "best practice" at the time. Chinese health authorities took the initiative to try out these unique responses, sometimes in the face of opposition from both domestic and foreign constituencies. The most notable example of this was the decision in 2004 actively to seek out people who had sold plasma in the mid-1990s, and to offer them HIV testing. The programme identified tens of thousands of people who needed HIV treatment, and successfully linked a high proportion of them with the healthcare services they needed. In some areas, social support for affected families and communities was also provided. Following the success of this programme, active testing strategies were expanded to other populations at high risk for HIV.

Another example of bold programming was the provision of methadone to drug users on a massive scale. Methadone programmes are promoted by HIV prevention specialists working with drug injectors in many countries, but they have met with staunch political resistance in some of the countries most in need of them – the most notable example being Russia. Unlike those countries, China put the health of its citizens first; it now provides treatment for some 200,000 heroin users, and has been rewarded with a steep drop in new HIV infections in this group.

Putting national needs first

In the early years of the HIV epidemic in China, much of the response was supported by loans or grants that came from outside the country. In many other lower- and middle-income countries, this led to a somewhat chaotic situation in which foreign donors (and sometimes even implementing NGOs) set their own priorities, often determined by their own institutional interests.

China did things differently. From the very start, almost all projects were discussed together with Chinese health authorities and researchers; those domestic authorities had a strong voice in directing funding to areas that would produce the greatest learning and potentially the greatest impact for the country. In addition, as it built up its own funding streams and programmes expanded, China took the international community at its word, and began to implement the principle of "Three Ones", in which foreign-supported programmes and data collection were integrated into a nationally led framework that prioritised the needs of China's citizens, rather than the interests of different international agencies.

The importance of political leadership

China's experience demonstrates very clearly indeed the importance of political leadership, not just at the highest level but also in areas most affected by this diverse epidemic. The response to HIV in China took off on a massive scale only after the country's highest leaders threw their weight behind prevention and care efforts. But even before that, significant successes had been achieved by enlightened and adventurous local administrators who witnessed the damage that AIDS was doing to individuals, families and communities in their area. These local officials encouraged experimentation which later provided the country's top leaders with evidence on which to base decisions that affected the nation as a whole.

A dedicated workforce

In the early years of the epidemic, HIV-related work was not popular. A few people chose the field out of personal conviction; many more were assigned the task simply because they were quite junior. One of them was Xi Chen, now a Deputy Director of Hunan provinces CDC, who was sent to work on AIDS as a new graduate, way back in the late 1980s. "AIDS was called plague of the century and super cancer so nobody wanted to do this work," he said. "Even I felt uneasy about it." Chen has been doing HIV-related work ever since. Many of the "AIDS Warriors" who took a personal interest in HIV at the start of the epidemic have stayed in this sector for their whole careers. This kind of experience and institutional memory is extraordinarily rare in public health services, especially in lower- and middle-income countries. It has built continuity and progressive learning into China's response, where in other settings people sometimes repeat past errors because nobody remembers that something has already been tried and found not to work.

The Chinese system has another advantage: the people who are active in health research are often also making decisions about service provision, and many go on to become senior policy makers themselves. This means that people who are best placed to learn from operations research and are most familiar with the situation on the ground are also in a position to take decisions that are based on strong evidence.

Challenges

As we've seen in the preceding chapters, China has fought many successful battles against HIV over the last three decades, but the war is by no means over. The country continues to face a number of challenges, some old and others new.

Enduring stigma: silence is deadly

Perhaps most intractable of the remaining challenges is the discrimination suffered by people living with HIV in China. The very government which passes laws to protect the rights of people with HIV continues to deny them employment. The very health authorities that have done so much to expand treatment for people with HIV also preside over a health service which turns infected people away from hospitals and refuses them surgery. Though the country's most senior leaders have tried to show their support for affected communities, their commitment often does not trickle down to other levels of government or society.

The stigma that seems to hang like a great cloud over the HIV-infected in China stands in the way of normalising the infection, of treating it like any other manageable, chronic condition. It also dissuades people from discussing their own infection, including with their own families and sex partners. With testing on the rise, more people than ever before know their own HIV status. But many continue to have unprotected sex, simply to avoid disclosing their own infection.

Some believe that the state should respond by criminalising this behaviour. Certainly, people who know they are infected should be supported in taking responsibility for their own actions and for the safety of their partners. However, experience in other countries suggests that criminalisation does very little to interrupt HIV transmission. Rather, it entrenches the very stigma that discourages open discussion and disclosure of HIV infection, while making contact tracing virtually impossible.

It is not just the virus itself that is stigmatised in China; it is the behaviours that spread it. Though sex is fundamental to human existence, many Chinese citizens would rather not discuss it openly. Parents and schools remain very resistant to the idea that young people should be taught about the mechanics of reproduction, let alone about wider topics such as sexuality. Taboos breed ignorance, ignorance breeds fear, fear breeds stigma and stigma breeds active discrimination. Young people, for their part, want to know about the changes their bodies are undergoing, about relationships, about love. Many Chinese teenagers turn to their peers or to the internet for information about these things; both sources are as likely to provide misinformation as to foster understanding.

A changing epidemic: gay men, sexual transmission

As other routes of HIV transmission are controlled, the importance of male–male sex in spreading the virus in China becomes more evident. This population presents very different challenges compared with those most affected earlier in the epidemic. Ending transmission to plasma sellers was relatively easy; it just required proper oversight of blood collection practices. Eliminating HIV transmission among drug injectors is also not too hard. Injectors do not generally want to share needles – they do so because they do not have easy, affordable and safe access to sterile equipment. Where that's provided, it will be used. Injectors who hope to overcome their addiction will also welcome substitute drugs such as methadone that they can take orally. Prevention interventions are also generally appreciated by women and men who sell sex. For them, the primary concern is not the distant prospect of HIV, but rather the far more immediate danger of other sexually transmitted infections (STIs). These interrupt work and put a dent in income; much better to use a condom than to lose money. If they do get infected, they want to get treated and back to work quickly, so the STI treatment services that also reduce the risk of HIV transmission are popular too. Clients are also often concerned about STIs, and are thus generally willing to use condoms.

In short, whether or not plasma sellers, drug injectors, sex workers and their clients have any interest in preventing HIV, they are largely happy to use the services that reduce their risk of infection.

The same is simply not true of gay men, nor, indeed of the non-commercial heterosexual couples who are also an increasingly large part of the epidemic in

China. In intimate relations, most people value the appearance of trust more highly than disease prevention, so it is far harder to persuade lovers to use condoms than it is to persuade sex workers and their clients. Channels of communication differ, too. Their behaviour may be frowned upon in some circles, but it is not illegal. They cannot be reached, as drug users and sex workers can be, through public security services or in rehabilitation settings. In the cities, this new generation of socially networked young people intent on individual expression are not particularly interested in listening to the injunctions of political leaders or in dancing to the tunes called by health officials.

A socially embedded approach

China has done a remarkable job of ramping up its health services to provide HIV testing and treatment services. Clinical prevention services, including methadone for drug injectors and antiretrovirals to prevent the transmission of HIV from pregnant women to their newborns, are now provided on a significant scale nationwide. For over five years, the 110,000 couples with one positive and one negative partner have also now had access to immediate treatment to reduce transmission within marriages. The further increase of testing and treatment among those at high risk may reduce onward transmission of HIV even more in the immediate future. But as Chapter 7 described, limited progress has been made in addressing the social, economic and cultural factors that shape behaviour and that put people at risk for HIV. Political and economic pressures to limit family size together with very strong cultural pressure to have a son have combined, for example, to create an imbalance in the sex ratio among people who are now coming of age sexually. It is not known whether that has contributed to the evident rise in same-sex relations between young men in China's cities, but it is perfectly plausible. What is clear is that these social drivers of risk are very deeply embedded and lie beyond the reach of health authorities. Addressing them will require commitment, effort and activity far beyond the nation's hospitals and health centres. These efforts will need to be resourced; as an increasing proportion of the HIV-specific budget is used up by treatment, it will be important to protect funding for programmes that prevent HIV both directly and indirectly, especially in the populations at highest risk.

Adapting for the future

China has a history of reacting pragmatically to overcome the hurdles to well-being thrown up by the HIV epidemic, particularly over the last decade. The strengths that allowed it to do this well have not disappeared. Addressing the challenges listed above will, however, require using those strengths in different ways.

Community engagement in the response

A changing epidemic, driven now by behaviours that are themselves shaped by a rapidly changing society, will require a new engagement by affected communities, and by society as a whole. This is not just about increasing access to individuals so that they can be tested for HIV and treated if necessary. It is not just about going around karaoke bars handing out leaflets and condoms. It is about encouraging communities to define their roles and take responsibility for their own well-being and destiny. Safe behaviours cannot be imposed by authorities; ultimately new community norms must be developed by the people who will adhere to them. As China HIV/AIDS Information Network's Lingping Cai says: "No one can control the development of society, you can't control the people's sex or desire to have sex, you can't control technology. But NGOs have the flexibility to help people to protect themselves in the way that people favour."

Experience in other countries suggests that it is possible, indeed even likely, that communities will come up with approaches to HIV prevention that differ from those promoted by health departments. Indeed, they may initially come up with approaches which don't directly address the virus at all, by working first to reduce discrimination based on sexual preference or to promote healthier lifestyles, for example. These may be the things that drive the social changes needed to support safer sexual behaviour in the medium term. They won't be achieved just by subcontracting community groups to deliver existing services to a larger number of people. They require genuine partnerships, and that implies a more equitable balance of influence in deciding what the priorities for action must be. As the WHO's

Bernhard Schwartländer said: "The funds are there for NGOs, and that's a huge step forward. What's missing right now is a platform through which NGOs can actually participate in decision-making."

Supporting community development is a relatively new experience for the Chinese authorities and the habit will not become entrenched overnight. The Chinese government, in common with almost every other government in the world, is wary of working with community groups in part because they aren't sure how to hold them accountable. That's especially a challenge at a time when the government is putting a strong emphasis on ensuring that public money is well spent, and that taxpayer-supported initiatives deliver results. Accountability is also important to the people whom community organisations claim to represent. Non-government groups, for their part, often don't have the experience necessary to follow the complex accounting procedures demanded of them, and many are not used to thinking about how the impact of their work can be measured. CDCs' officers can help them in this task by sharing data and information about the local epidemic, but a culture of information exchange is not yet well established.

There is no doubt that communities will have to step up and take more responsibility for their own health and welfare if the current wave of HIV infection is to be overcome. This is especially true of gay men, both young and old, but experience from other countries suggests that when sex workers and drug injectors come together, they can also greatly improve their own welfare. Both groups are currently massively under-served by China's nascent non-government sector.

It is clear that authorities at the local, provincial and central levels want to control the HIV epidemic; it's also clear that where that control involves changes in community norms around something as intimate as sex, they need to work in partnership with those most affected. The existing fund to support community groups will, for the first time, allow salaries to be paid, which means that people will be able to earn a decent living by supporting their communities. This will contribute to the professionalization of community organisations. As experience with using these funding channels grows and government and non-government groups grow more comfortable working together, trust will develop, genuine partnerships will be more likely to flourish, and HIV prevention efforts more likely to succeed.

Breaking the silence

The Chinese leadership has made its commitment to supporting those living with HIV very clear indeed. However, the enduring discrimination against people living with HIV in China will continue unless health service providers and government employees at all levels of society share that commitment. China has done well to create a supporting legal framework for people with HIV, but without enforcement, the laws have no value. China has made a huge financial and logistical commitment to provide treatment to prolong the lives of people with HIV, only to allow them to be continually robbed of their dignity. To meet the commitments it has made in international forums, as well as the pledges that China's senior leaders have made to the people they govern, officials at all levels will have to turn their attention and energy to enforcing anti-discrimination laws, and to sanctioning those who violate them.

Discrimination is fed by stigma, and the stigma surrounding HIV continues to be fed by statements and campaigns that demonise the behaviours that spread the virus. This simply entrenches negative attitudes towards people who are infected. But it doesn't seem to have much effect on risk behaviours themselves. There's no indication that Chinese citizens are losing their appetite for commercial sex, and behavioural surveillance suggests that both extramarital sex and sex between men are on the rise. These societal changes follow a pattern also seen recently in many other Asian countries. However, they are rarely talked about, and young people are left without reliable information about sex and sexuality.

China's ministry of education has now recognised this gap in information, which has contributed to a steep rise in HIV infections among (mostly male) college students across China. But at the local level, educators sometimes react to the issue of increasing sexual expression among young people simply by denying it. In an effort to undermine this denial, local health departments have now been tasked with keeping education authorities up to date with what's really going on in their local epidemics. No concrete steps have yet been taken to increase sex education in primary or secondary schools. But in a programme backed by the nation's First Lady, Peng Liyuan, college students in some 40 universities nationwide are now being supported to discuss HIV with their peers, to answer questions about the virus, and to offer HIV tests.

90-90-90

New initiatives do not imply that past successes should be abandoned. Though it's evident that China needs to expand its approach to HIV beyond the biomedical, it will continue to strive to ensure that people with HIV get the treatment they need. China was among the very first countries to formally adopt the '90-90-90' targets set by UNAIDS in 2014: 90% of infected people should know their status, 90% of diagnosed cases should receive antiretroviral medication, and for 90% of those on therapy, the virus should fall to levels undetectable using standards tests.

These numerical targets are intended merely as calls to action. They are all dependent on the estimated number of people living with HIV, which, as we saw in Chapter 5, is in itself an imprecise number. China's efforts are driven less by a numerical target than by a commitment to reach as many people as possible with testing and treatment services. China's current official estimates indicate that close to 70% of those infected have been diagnosed. Some people who think they may be at risk are probably reluctant to test because they don't believe results will be kept confidential. To overcome this barrier, China will promote the use of self-testing. More service provision by community based groups who have the freedom to work with greater independence from the health authorities is also likely to improve customer-centred service, encouraging those who test positive in home testing to seek care.

Two recent policy changes will contribute greatly to increasing the proportion of diagnosed people who take medicine to control the virus. The first is a decision, announced in June 2016, to drop any biological thresholds for treatment. Until then, people had to get tested to see whether their CD4 blood cell count was below 500 per millilitre before they could be treated. Though the "one-stop shop" services reduced drop-out, some continued to slip out of the health services at this point, and the threshold itself reduced the proportion of those diagnosed who were eligible for treatment to just 78%. The second change that should boost treatment numbers is a long-awaited commitment to provide new medicines, including combination pills which make it far easier for people to take their medicines as they should. The limited range of medicines available and the failure to switch to newer formulations with fewer side-effects has contributed to slow uptake of antiretroviral therapy in China. Newer, easier-to-take drugs should encourage more newly diagnosed people to embrace the opportunity offered by treatment, especially if they can easily get hold of those drugs wherever they are in the country. Wider access to more convenient drugs will help people to take their medications more consistently, while a wider variety will provide more options for rapid switching if people develop side-effects or if the virus becomes resistant to the drugs they are taking. Both of these things will improve viral suppression, contributing to progress towards the third target. The drive to ensure that targets are met will require more regular monitoring of viral loads, which will have an important benefit for clients because it helps doctors to spot potential treatment failure sooner.

The journey continues

HIV has taught China a lot over the last 30 years. It reminded the nation that it was not isolated from the world, that physical borders are not effective barriers to virus, nor indeed to technological and social changes. The fate of tens of thousands of people who sold their plasma and became infected with HIV underlined the serious human consequences that sometimes accompany the headlong rush for economic growth. Denial was shown to be not only useless but also damaging. The power of real political commitment to drive effective change, on the other hand, has been demonstrated very clearly.

Many lessons are equally valuable for other countries, too. The importance of understanding the specific features of local HIV epidemics and of building up a strong evidence base have been underlined by China's experience. A willingness to take risks, to seek pragmatic solutions and to adapt to changing circumstances has been the bedrock of the nation's success.

As long as that pragmatism and flexibility continue to underpin the response to HIV, China's government and its citizens will be in a strong position to face the next decade with confidence, knowing that they will be able to work together to limit the number of new infections and to improve the well-being of people who live with HIV.

Appendix

HIV in China: 30 Years in Numbers

Elizabeth Pisani and Zunyou Wu

As we have seen throughout this book, the HIV epidemic in China developed in ways that were neither simple nor predictable. The virus has spread differently in different parts of this vast country. The groups most affected have changed over time, too, not only because successful prevention programmes are now in place for some groups but also because of the radical social change which China has undergone over the course of the epidemic.

This chapter is designed to be a stand-alone summary of the entire epidemic; it thus repeats the broad narrative of the earlier chapters, but focuses particularly on the data that underpin the changes described earlier. Unless otherwise noted, all data in this chapter come from China CDC's National Centre for AIDS/STD Control and Prevention.

The evolving epidemic

In retrospect, it seems likely that a handful of people were infected in the early 1980s because they were given imported blood products that had not been adequately screened. The first person known to have AIDS in China, however, was a United States citizen who died of the disease in 1985. At the time, China was newly emerging from a period of relative isolation. The behaviours known to spread HIV – drug injection, sex between men and commercial sex – were believed not to exist in the country. As long as blood products and foreigners carrying the virus could be excluded, Chinese health officials felt, there was no real risk of an epidemic developing in China. Imported blood products were banned just three months after the first recorded AIDS death, and foreigners planning to live in China were screened for the virus.

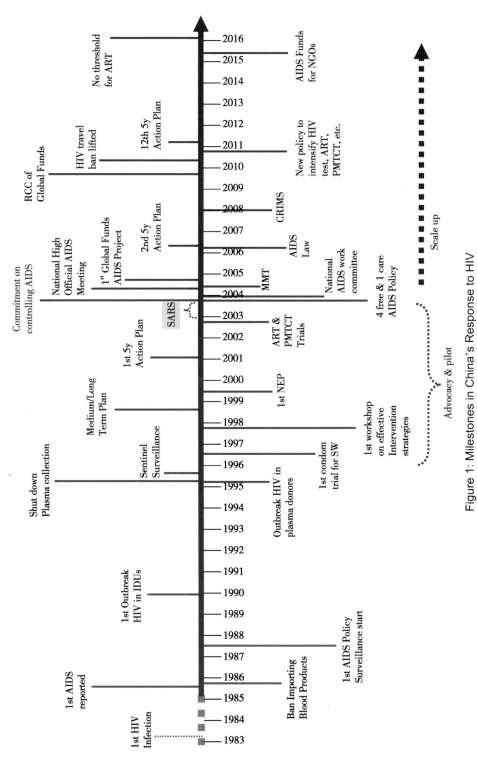

Figure 1: Milestones in China's Response to HIV

Drug injecting spreads HIV in south-western China

The authorities were thus caught unawares when HIV surfaced in the most unlikely place: not among gay men or sex workers in big cities, but in isolated villages in one of the remotest corners of Yunnan province, in south-western China. Though public security officials had known that heroin was seeping across the border from Myanmar, and was increasingly being injected by some people in rural Yunnan, they did not share that information with health officials. It was almost by accident that an epidemiologist who specialised in hepatitis in the local disease prevention station discovered an outbreak of HIV among drug injectors in detention: two in five of the drug users she tested for HIV were positive.

Public health officials in Beijing, working with public security authorities, quickly put in place HIV surveillance among drug injectors in all the regions where they were then known to exist, mostly in western and south-western China. They found no sign at the time that the virus had spread beyond Yunnan. It was not until 1995 that injectors were found to be infected with HIV in the westernmost province of Xinjiang, as well as in Yunnan's neighbour, Sichuan. Over the first 20 years of the epidemic in China, people who injected drugs accounted for 44% of all the HIV cases identified in the country. If the cases known to result from the sale of blood and plasma are excluded, the proportion rises to some 63%. This probably overstates the true proportion, simply because, historically, people who took illegal drugs in China were channelled into detoxification centres. That means they were more likely than non-injectors to be tested for HIV, and thus more likely to be identified as a case and reported to the health authorities. Nonetheless, there is no doubt that sharing needles during drug injection was the most important driver of HIV infection in the early phases of China's epidemic.

Plasma sales drive a second wave of HIV

Public health officials suffered a second major shock in the mid-1990s, when companies screening blood plasma in Shanghai began to identify HIV-positive specimens collected from commercial donors in rural areas in central China.

People collecting the blood locally were slow to understand the significance of the test results that were reported back to them. The local CDC office in Anhui province at first assumed that the infections must have been acquired sexually. As they investigated further, however, it became apparent that people were contracting HIV during the process of plasma collection itself. The central government moved rapidly to shut down the plasma collection stations that provided an important source of income for poorer people in the industrially under-developed provinces of central China. They did not, however, anticipate that plasma collectors would simply shift to taking blood directly from peasants in villages. This practice, which included re-injecting people with pooled red blood cells so that they could give blood again sooner, continued for at least a year after the outbreak was first identified. To make matters worse, blood used in transfusions by local hospitals was not regularly screened at the time. Because of that, many people who had never sold blood themselves were infected while seeking healthcare.

One survey from an academic paper published by respected Chinese scientists carried out at the time in three counties in Anhui province suggested that in some villages up to one in nine plasma sellers was infected, but local officials across the affected areas were reluctant to make the information public.[72]It was not until around five years later, when large numbers of people began to sicken and die, that the history of the outbreak became more widely known. The true extent of the HIV infections among this population in Henan, Anhui and other areas of central China will probably never be known, but it is clear that the tragedy had an important, if belated, impact on the response to the HIV epidemic in China.

Tracking the path of the virus

Other parts of the epidemic were better understood as they unfolded, in large part because of the country's growing sentinel surveillance system. In sentinel surveillance, blood samples are taken from people who are visiting a facility such as a clinic for pregnant women, a clinic treating sexually transmitted infections or a drug treatment clinic. These samples are often taken to screen for other conditions such as syphilis or hepatitis. During the sentinel surveillance period, blood is also screened for HIV. This provides a robust idea of HIV prevalence – the proportion currently infected – within the population represented by those visiting the clinic.

Though China's HIV sentinel surveillance system was not fully standardised until 2010, meaning that data from earlier years were not always exactly comparable, all high-prevalence and many lower-prevalence areas had functioning sentinel surveillance sites (overseen by national and local authorities) in both female sex workers and drug users from 1995. That year, there were a total of 42 sites. Eight of them collected blood samples from drug users, and 13 from female sex workers. The remainder of the sites took blood from two groups expected to represent people with risky sexual behaviour: long-distance truck drivers and patients of clinics treating sexually transmitted infections (STIs). Over time, the system expanded geographically and other populations were added, including, from 2002, a site representing gay men. Since 2010, there have been 1,888 sentinel sites giving comparable data over time. Of those, 303 are among drug injectors, 520 among sex workers and 108 among men who have sex with men.

Analysis of different sub-types of HIV as well as phylogenetics– which uses gene sequencing to track the spread of a the virus from one person to another – suggests that the virus that spread so quickly among plasma sellers in central China in the mid-1990s had in fact been passed on from drug injectors in Yunnan province.[21,73] The spread of HIV through injecting networks was accelerated as China's economy boomed and new roads and other transport options allowed people and drugs to move much more freely. HIV took six years to spread from the then-isolated south-western corner of Yunnan to neighbouring Sichuan and to Xinjiang. In the following five years the virus spread into another 23 provinces, bringing the total number of provinces reporting HIV among drug injectors to 26. It took just another two years to find its way into injecting communities in the final seven provinces and autonomous regions; by 2002, HIV was recorded in sentinel surveillance among drug injectors in every province in China.

Limited spread through commercial sex

By 2002, more than one out of every two drug injectors was found to be infected with HIV in many independent studies in western and south-western China. A recent review of several hundred studies together with sentinel surveillance data from the time suggest that one out of every ten drug injectors was infected across the nation as a whole.[74] Some female injectors financed their drug purchases by selling sex, and in surveys of risk behaviour among male injectors, a high proportion also reported buying sex. On top of that, condom use among drug injectors on both the sex worker and the client side was lower than among men and women who did not use drugs, which of course meant that there was a high risk that the virus would pass into commercial sex networks.

And indeed it did, although it was only in the areas that already had highly developed drug-driven epidemics that HIV among sex workers became well established, reaching around 2% in south-western China – four times higher than in other areas of the country. Elsewhere in the country, less than one female sex worker in 200 was infected with HIV.

Infection rates among women who sell sex probably stayed relatively low for a number of reasons. Condoms are actively promoted among sex workers to avoid sexually transmitted infections other than HIV, and condom use is the norm for clients who buy sex from women working in nightclubs, bars, karaoke lounges and beauty shops (although men who buy sex from women working on the streets are far less likely to use condoms). In addition, turnover among sex workers is high. This limits potential exposure; it may also mean that women who became infected while they sold sex are no longer reflected in the statistics because they have since moved on to other occupations.

HIV takes off among gay men

By the mid-2000s, China's epidemic was undergoing another big change. More and more cases were being registered among young men who had contracted the infection while having unprotected anal sex with other men. The trends in HIV infection rates over the past decade and a half in China are shown in Figure 2. The data come from sentinel surveillance sites that sometimes differed from year to year up until 2010, when the system was standardised. However they are comparable enough to give an idea of the broad changes in each group.

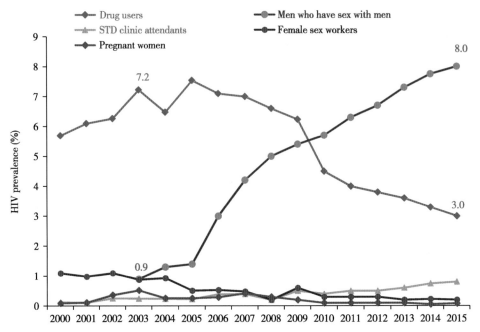

Figure 2: HIV prevalence in different sentinel surveillance populations, China, 2000–2015, all national sites

Two of these changes are particularly striking. The first is the rather steep fall in HIV infection among people who take drugs. The second, more shocking change is the steep rise in the proportion of gay and bisexual men who are living with HIV. Both of these trends have continued during the years in which there has been no change to sentinel sites, suggesting that they are unlikely to be an artefact of changes in sampling strategies.

The falling prevalence among drug users is the more easily explained of the two trends, with two major factors contributing to the lower rates. The first is a likely change in the people who are tested. The surveillance population is not restricted to injectors, so HIV among people who take opiates and other drugs orally will also be reflected in these data. If trends in drug use change, with methamphetamines and other drugs that are swallowed or sniffed becoming more popular relative to drugs that are injected, then the tested population will include new users who were never at risk through injection. At the same time, many of the older injectors infected early in the epidemic will have died and thus also dropped out of the pool of people at sentinel sites. The second factor pushing down HIV rates among drug users over time is the success of prevention efforts, including the provision of sterile injecting equipment and methadone. Easy access to clean needles and syringes greatly reduces the needle sharing that spreads HIV. Oral methadone as a substitute for injected heroin, on the other hand, helps drug users to stop buying and injecting heroin or other opiates. This also cuts down the likelihood that they will share needles and contract or pass on a blood-borne virus such as HIV or Hepatitis C, without necessarily requiring that they immediately take the harder step of giving up addictive drugs. There is very little evidence that the practice of obliging drug users to attend detoxification programmes reduces substance abuse or the harms associated with it; however, as long as the policy exists, it represents an opportunity to link drug users into other health and welfare programmes, including HIV prevention or treatment.

As the left-hand graph in Figure 3 shows, newly diagnosed HIV cases among male drug injectors have fallen dramatically in the years since HIV testing has been actively promoted in populations at high risk, confirming the trends seen in sentinel surveillance.

In 2011, newly diagnosed cases in men who injected drugs and men who had sex with other men – each represented by the lightest-shaded of the areas on the graph in Figure 3 – stood at similar levels in 2010; around 10,000 new diagnoses in each population.But the trends then diverged. While newly reported cases among drug injectors fell in each successive year, cases contracted during sex between men shot upwards, reaching over 32,600 by 2015. Most drug injectors with newly diagnosed HIV are between 25 and 45 years old. Among gay men, on the other hand, there's a steep peak at ages below 30. Educational level doesn't seem to provide much protection. Figure 4 shows the transmission route for all people who reported being in college when they were first diagnosed with HIV from 2011 to 2015. Newly diagnosed

HIV infections among female college students remained rare throughout that time, never exceeding 70 infections in a year. Among male students, however, infections were more than 30times higher, and they tripled in just that four-year period. The proportion of those men admitting to being infected in sex with another man rose from 75% in 2011 to 85% in 2015. While the absolute numbers are tiny relative to the millions of young people studying in China's universities, the trends are clearly very worrying.

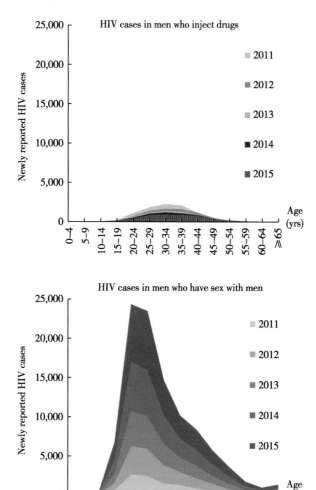

Figure 3: Newly reported HIV cases among male drug injectors and men who have sex with men in China, 2011–2015

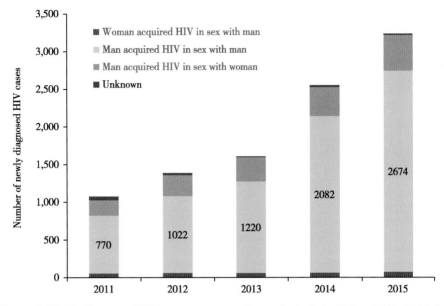

Figure 4: Newly diagnosed HIV cases among college students in China, 2011–2015, by reported mode of transmission

As Chapter 7 noted, there are several reasons for this extraordinarily rapid rise in HIV infections contracted during sex between men. The greater social acceptability of same-sex behaviour, a general increase in the accessibility of gay-focused entertainment venues even in smaller cities, and above all the explosion of social and sexual networking through the internet and smart phones: all these have greatly increased the opportunities for Chinese men wanting to find male sex partners, compared with just a decade ago. The result: in that decade, the proportion of newly reported HIV infections that were clearly acquired during sex between men ballooned 10-fold, from 2.5% in 2006 to 28.3% in 2015.

One of the most worrying features of the HIV epidemic among gay men in China is that it is spreading geographically far more than any previous epidemic has done. While HIV infections among drug injectors and sex workers are found around the country, rather a small proportion of sentinel sites register particularly high infection rates. HIV prevalence exceeds 5% in just 19% of sentinel sites among drug injectors nationwide, and those are clustered in the south-west and far west of the country. Among sex workers,

HIV prevalence remains below 1% in all but 6% of sites – mostly in the same areas where many drug users are infected. Among gay men, on the other hand, 66% of sentinel surveillance sites are already showing HIV prevalence at over 5%–fully two-thirds. Many of those are on the eastern seaboard and in other areas until now little affected by HIV.

Heading for parallel epidemics?

It is almost as though China is now experiencing two parallel but largely separate epidemics. One, in large cities in areas previously little affected by HIV, is driven overwhelmingly by sex between young men. The other, in the west and south-western parts of China that have been coping with HIV for two decades, shows a much more even balance between infections acquired in homosexual and heterosexual partnerships.

Figure 5 shows the remarkable difference in the sex ratio of newly diagnosed infections in two indicative areas: Beijing, representing the "new" epidemic, and Yunnan, home to the oldest indigenous epidemic in China.

Although it has done more than almost any other part of China to expand its HIV prevention services, including access to testing for those at highest risk, Yunnan continues to diagnose a significant number of new cases each year. But Beijing is catching up, at least as far as infections among men are concerned. The capital diagnosed more men than the south-western province did in 2015, relative to its population size. However, new HIV infections among women in the Chinese capital remain extraordinarily rare: just over 100 women were diagnosed in 2015, compared with close to 3,900 in Yunnan (which has about three times as many residents as Beijing). Overall, the sex ratio of infection in Beijing was 28:1. In Yunnan, it was less than 2:1.

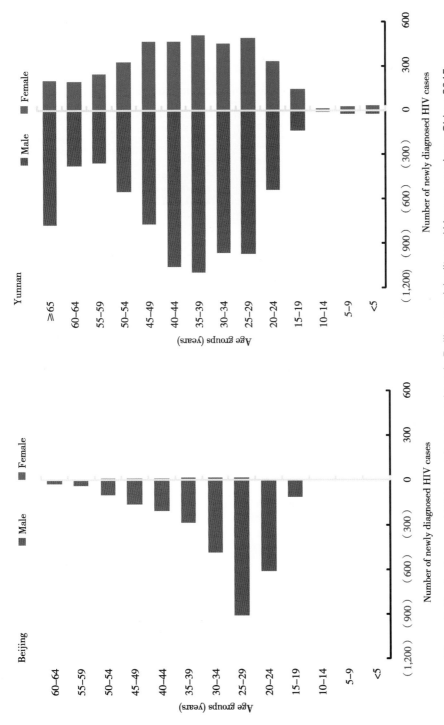

Figure 5: Newly diagnosed HIV cases by age and sex in Beijing municipality and Yunnan province, China, 2015

Uncertainly over growing heterosexual transmission

A question mark remains over the extent of heterosexual HIV transmission in China. In 2015, 95% of newly diagnosed infections in women and 58% in men were reported as having been acquired during sex between a man and a woman – a more detailed picture is given in Figure 6.

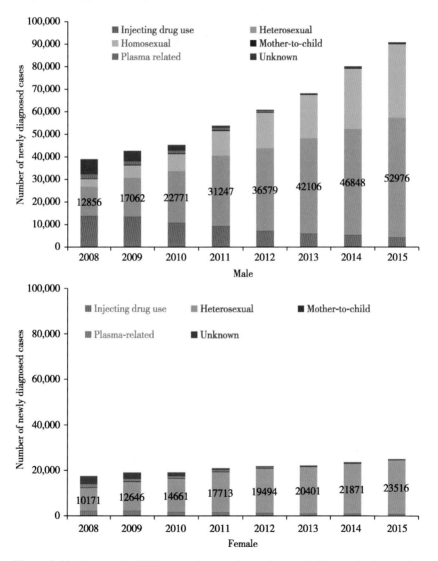

Figure 6: Newly reported HIV cases by gender and reported transmission route, China, 2008–2015

These infections can be divided into three broad types: those acquired within marriage or another live-in partnership, those acquired when selling or buying sex, and those acquired in sex with a casual partner, including transient girlfriends and boyfriends. Looking in greater detail at infections reported to be acquired heterosexually, we see significant differences between men and women.

HIV transmission between husband and wife

Fewer than 2,000 men newly diagnosed with HIV in 2015 who reported acquiring HIV heterosexually said that they were infected by their wives. Over 6,300 women reported being infected by their husbands, however. (That's 4% of male heterosexual infections, and 27% of female heterosexual infections respectively.) Just 653 of them occurred in couples known by health services to be sero-discordant, with one HIV-infected and one uninfected spouse. This suggests that efforts to reduce onward transmission of HIV within marriages by ensuring that the HIV-infected partner is treated and is thus less infectious are succeeding. While some of the infections reported as occurring within marriage may have been misreported to avoid admitting to extramarital sex, the substantial difference in the numbers also suggests that there are still many discordant couples unknown to the health services.

Prominent among these may be married couples in which the husband acquired HIV during sex with another man. In an investigation carried out in 2013, over a third of men newly diagnosed with an HIV infection contracted from another man, reported having a female partner. Similarly, in a recent study of over 1,500 men attending a gay sauna in the north-eastern city of Tianjin, nearly a third reported that they had had unprotected sex with a female partner in the preceding six months.[75] Perhaps reflecting the less tolerant social norms of their younger years, older gay men are far more likely to be married. In a five-city study of men who have sex with men conducted in 2013, 82% of men over 50 reported being married, compared with 57% of those aged 30–49 and just 7% of the under 30s.[76] These men are often not open with their wives about their homosexual partners. If they know their HIV status, they may very well hide it from their wives, at the same time avoiding disclosing their marital status to health authorities for fear of being "outed".

If women became infected during sex with husbands or boyfriends who also have sex with other men, their cases would be included in the spousal or casually acquired heterosexual infections reported above. In the long run, however, the most effective way to reduce these sorts of infections among women is of course to prevent their male partners becoming infected via sex with other men. In other words, effective prevention programmes for gay and bisexual men will reduce heterosexual transmission, also.

Heterosexual transmission outside marriage

Perhaps surprisingly, over 60% of heterosexually infected women said they were infected with HIV in sex with a man who was not their husband or regular partner. Men, on the other hand, were less likely to report casual sex as a source of heterosexual infection. Over half of all men heterosexually infected in 2015 said they acquired HIV from a sex worker (53% in all), while another 40% said they were exposed to HIV by their girlfriends or casual lovers. That is 28,000 newly diagnosed HIV infections among clients of commercial sex workers in 2015, compared with fewer than 2,500 new diagnoses among sex workers themselves – despite very widespread testing among women who sell sex. Because female sex workers serve many male clients, the absolute number of men infected in commercial sex with women is usually higher than the number of women infected. Epidemics driven by commercial sex generally record sex ratios of infection of about 4:1, so the ratio among new diagnoses in China seems unusually high.

Part of this may be explained because men who were infected many years ago are just now being diagnosed (see "Viagra ™ Generation", below). But it seems likely, also, that a significant portion of the HIV infections reported by men as being acquired heterosexually are actually acquired during sex with other men. Though male–male sex is increasingly easily available in China, it remains stigmatised, especially among older generations. Rather than admit to homosexual behaviour, some men may prefer to report the more socially acceptable behaviour of buying sex from a woman. One special study carried out among men who reported heterosexual transmission in 2014 to evaluate this issue found that 15% of such cases were actually the result of homosexual contact, rather than heterosexual transmission.

By simply calculating the proportion of new cases reported as acquired in commercial sex at a more usual ratio of 4:1 compared with sex worker diagnoses, we can get an extremely rough idea of the number of homosexually acquired infections among men that might have been misreported as heterosexual: some 18,000 in 2015. Adjusting likely routes of transmission using that crude estimate, we find that 57% of newly diagnosed infections in men could have been acquired during sex between men in China (and 38% heterosexually). This would almost exactly reverse the proportions shown in Figure 6, which indicated that only 36% were acquired homosexually, and 58% heterosexually.

The Viagra™ Generation?

One interesting feature of the current epidemic is the age distribution in newly-reported HIV infections. Figure 7 shows newly-reported infections in 2015 for all of China by gender and age group. It is hard not to notice the remarkably high number of newly-identified cases of HIV infection among older people, especially older men. In 2015, almost a quarter of men newly-identified as HIV-positive were aged over 60, compared with just two percent in 2006.

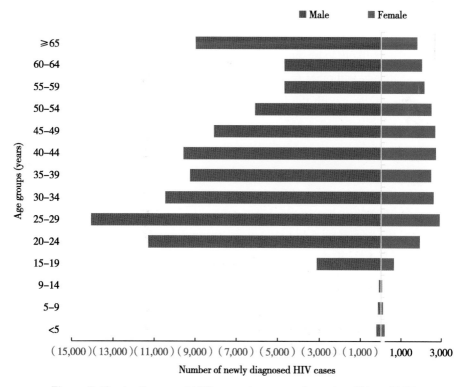

Figure 7: Newly diagnosed HIV cases by age and gender, China, 2015

There are several possible reasons for this. One is the age of the epidemic itself: some of these men may have been infected much earlier in China's epidemic, simply ageing with the virus. A second possibility is that these men belong to the "Viagra™ Generation"– the wide availability of drugs to treat erectile dysfunction has allowed them to extend their sexual activity and their exposure to risk. A third possibility, perhaps overlapping with the second, is that technology and social change has allowed older men who were never before able to access sex with other men to find commercial or casual partners of their own gender, from a pool that is now unfortunately much affected by HIV.

A more detailed examination of individual-level data suggests that the first of these reasons is the most probable. Most of the men first diagnosed when they are over 60 have CD4 cell counts well under 600 per millilitre, suggesting that they have been living with HIV for some years. It is probable that many of them are only diagnosed in their later years because the ageing process (and in some cases their advancing HIV infection) is bringing them into contact with medical services for the first time in many years. As routine testing of people in healthcare settings expands, women are more likely to be diagnosed earlier in the course of their infection, simply because pregnancy and other reproductive health issues tend to provide women with more routine contacts with the health services in their early adult years, compared with men.

Funding increases by leaps and bounds

Just as HIV prevention has evolved over time in China, so has treatment. As Chapter 7 described, this required a huge financial commitment on the part of the Chinese government. Figure 8 shows just how much the country now spends. The first significant contribution by the Chinese government was CNY100 million in 2001; around US$14 million at the time. By 2015, China was spending CNY3.7 billion – US$600 million at 2015 exchange rates. By 2015, some 42% of that money was spent on treatment, and another quarter on preventing transmission of HIV from pregnant women to their infants.

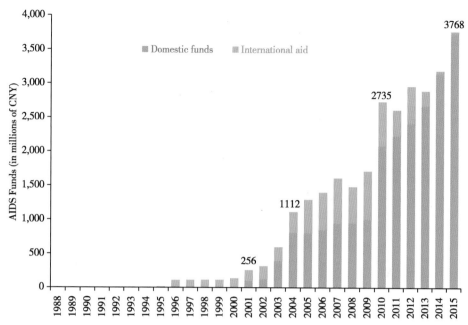

Figure 8: Spending on HIV-related treatment and care by source of funding,
China, 1988–2015

Ramping up testing and treatment

The watershed moment that led to this huge increase was surely in late 2003, when the government committed to making antiretroviral treatment and necessary social care available and affordable to all citizens. The logistical challenges alone were formidable; the first challenge was to increase the proportion of people who knew they were infected; that meant that HIV testing services needed to be made much more widely available. As Figure 9 shows, that happened very quickly. By 2004, China already carried out just under 20 million HIV tests a year; by 2015, the figure was seven times as high.

These tests are provided in a wide variety of different settings. Some of them, such as routine testing of all pregnant women, yield very few positive results relative to the huge numbers of tests undertaken; as Table 1 shows, of close to 19 million pregnant women screened for HIV in China in 2015, fewer than one in 10,000 was confirmed to have a previously unknown HIV infection. Perhaps surprisingly given the history of the epidemic in China, the lowest infection rates are among blood donors, including paid plasma donors. This reflects the very strong safety measures now applied to blood donors. Any person who has previously screened positive for HIV is not permitted to give blood again, and newly identified infections in this group are now rare. The highest proportion of previously undiagnosed infections was found among the spouses of people known to be HIV-infected. This confirms the value of contact tracing as an effective method of identifying people who may be in need of HIV-related treatment and care.

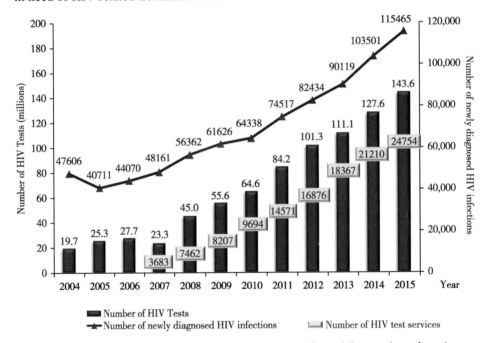

Figure 9: The number of HIV tests undertaken annually and the number of newly diagnosed infections, China, 2004–2015

Table 1: Number of HIV tests undertaken in different populations in China in 2015, with number and proportion positive

Population being tested for HIV	HIV tests	New HIV diagnoses	New diagnoses per 10,000 tests
Surgery	44,990,604	13,498	3.00
Transfusion	6,591,229	974	1.48
STD clinic attendants	2,503,842	6739	26.91
Other patients	30,335,464	37,381	12.32

(Table 1 continued)

Population being tested for HIV	HIV tests	New HIV diagnoses	New diagnoses per 10,000 tests
Antenatal Care	18,875,004	1665	0.88
Subtotal, medical services	**103,296,143**	**60,257**	**5.83**
Pre-marital care	6,518,088	2640	4.05
Voluntary counselling & testing	2,456,330	33,423	136.07
HIV+ individuals spouses	45,668	3852	843.48
Children of HIV+ women	6,417	259	403.62
Occupational exposure	15,209	5	3.29
Person in entertainment places	1,307,214	396	3.03
Paid plasma/blood donors	8,205,738	165	0.20
Voluntary plasma/blood donors	11,864,035	2769	2.33
Entry/exit border	710,107	280	3.94
New recruit for soldier	374,267	122	3.26
Drug users in detention centres	339,838	1647	48.46
Female sex workers in detention	15,794	70	44.32
Other detainees	1,394,661	2523	18.09
Special survey	2,714,989	3560	13.11
Others	4,318,619	3497	8.10
Total	**143,583,117**	**115,465**	**8.04**

The huge expansion of testing resulted in a huge expansion of people diagnosed as HIV-infected who were in need of care. That in turn required care services to be ramped up. By 2015, there were 4,226 health facilities across 2,415 counties of China providing antiretroviral treatment to patients with HIV. Just a decade after the commitment was made to provide treatment to those who needed it, close to nine out of every ten patients known to be eligible for treatment in China were in regular contact with the health services. The number of patients receiving treatment increased from fewer than 20,000 in 2005 to over 382,000 in 2015, as Figure 10 illustrates – over 85% of those known to be eligible.

As we saw in Chapter 6, until 2016, no one was considered eligible for treatment without a confirmed, positive HIV test *and* a CD4 cell count that indicated a certain level of disease progression. At first, this proved a major obstacle to getting people into treatment – people were dropping out at every stage. Then the "one-stop shop" described in Chapter 6 was tried. Together with other efforts by health authorities, expanding that new system has improved the situation dramatically.

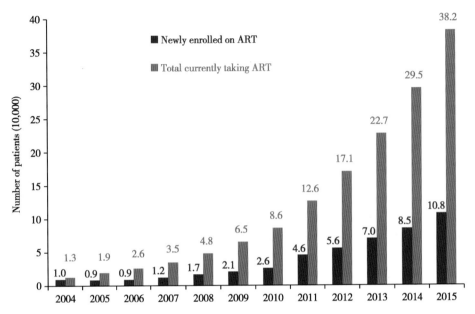

Figure 10: Number of patients starting antiretroviral therapy (ART) and number currently on treatment, China, 2004–2015

By 2012, the proportion of people screening positive who did not go on to get a confirmatory test had more than halved to 15% in hospital settings; it was slightly higher at 20% in the community health centres where offers of HIV testing are not yet routine.[46] And as Figure 11 shows, the proportion of people getting a CD4 test within the target period of two weeks after confirmatory testing shot up from just 11% in 2006 to 65% in 2015. Since 2013, some 86% of people with newlyconfirmed HIV diagnoses have had a CD4 test within six months of HIV diagnosis.

Overall, these efforts at expanding both the reach and quality of treatment have had a dramatic effect on death rates among people with HIV in China. Figure 12 illustrates this: as treatment rises among those who need it, death rates drop, not just in the population of eligible cases overall, but even among people who are on treatment. Though challenges remain, these data are a beacon of great hope.

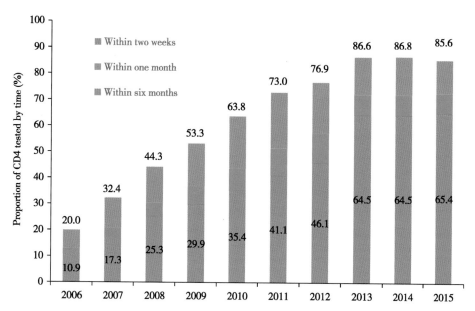

Figure 11: Percentage of people newly diagnosed with HIV who get CD4 tests, by time since confirmed HIV diagnosis. China, 2006–2015

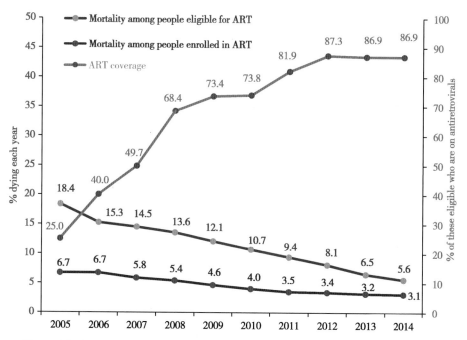

Figure 12: Percentage of those eligible for antiretroviral therapy (ART) who are on treatment. Annual mortality among all people eligible, and those on treatment, China, 2005–2014

In 2016, China eliminated the CD4 threshold as a condition for access to antiretrovirals. It is also trying to create opportunities to refashion care more closely to meet the needs of patients, rather than to conform to the habits of service providers. These challenges will be best met if China is able simultaneously to whittle away the considerable stigma which HIV patients continue to face within the health system itself.

What is next?

While China's progress in tackling its HIV epidemic has been remarkable, there is always room for improvement. To seize every opportunity for better prevention and care, it is important to understand the evolving epidemic. China's ever-improving surveillance systems and body of research is helping to do just that. Uncertainties will always remain, but pinpointing the exact source of the many infections reported as "heterosexual" is less important than understanding the overall picture as the country faces its fourth decade with HIV. It is a picture of increasing complexity.

China's approach to reducing HIV transmission in groups previously very much at risk has been reassuringly effective. New HIV infections resulting from blood products have been reduced to a handful each year at most. Though it is difficult to infer trends accurately from case report data because they depend in part on who is getting tested, case reports together with sentinel surveillance strongly suggest that new infections among drug users continue to fall, and HIV prevalence remains very low among women who sell sex in most of the country. Widespread partner testing and treatment are limiting transmission within heterosexual couples, also.

As the tide of infections in the groups once most at risk recedes, the rocks that represent ongoing HIV prevention and care challenges are exposed. The most obvious challenge in China, described in some detail in Chapter 7, is now in preventing the further spread of HIV among gay and behaviourally bisexual men. The gay community itself will without doubt have to lead involvement in HIV prevention; this challenges the traditionally rather top-down model of service implementation within the Chinese health system.

Additional challenges are presented by the dispersal of heterosexual risk away from the easily accessed commercial sphere and through more informal networks. HIV has never taken off among heterosexuals engaging in premarital or casual extramarital sex in any Asian or indeed any industrialised country, and there is no reason to believe that it might do so in China. However, because of the sheer size of the population, extremely low rates of transmission can still translate into a large number of women and men in need of care. These people don't belong to any obvious "high risk group", so it won't be easy to identify them in a cost-effective way.

These challenges are not small. However, as we hope this book has shown, China has a strong track record of trying out different and sometimes daring approaches, and of evaluating them honestly. Those that work are replicated quickly, and on a grand scale. These qualities should enable China to overcome the obstacles thrown up by the ever-changing HIV epidemic in its fourth decade and beyond.

References

1. Zhang W. China's Journey fighting AIDS – participant stories. Beijing: People's Medical Publishing House; 2015.

2. Macartney J. Chinese authorities ban sex with foreigners to stop AIDS. United Press International. Beijing; 1987 Sep 29.

3. Sullivan SG, Wu Z. Rapid scale up of harm reduction in China. International Journal of Drug Policy. 2007 Mar;18(2):118–28.

4. UNAIDS. HIV/AIDS: China's Titanic Peril, 2002. Update of the AIDS Situation and Needs Assessment Report. Beijing: June; 2002.

5. Shi L, Wang J, Liu Z, Stevens L, Sadler A, Ness P, et al. Blood donor management in China. Transfusion Medicine and Hemotherapy. 2014;41(4):273–82.

6. Bandurski D, Hala M. Investigative journalism in China: Eight cases in Chinese watchdog journalism. Hong Kong: Hong Kong University Press; 2010.

7. Yan J, Xiao S, Zhou L, Tang Y, Xu G, Luo D, et al. A social epidemiological study on HIV/AIDS in a village of Henan Province, China. AIDS Care. 2013;25(3):302–8.

8. Wu Z, Rou K, Detels R. Prevalence of HIV infection among former commercial plasma donors in rural eastern China. Health Policy and Planning. 2001;16(1):41–6.

9. Wu Z, Dong N, Guo W. Discovery and control of the HIV/AIDS epidemic among plasma donors in China. In: Li L, Zhan S, editors. Epidemiological Research Cases in China. Beijing: People's Medical Publishing House; 2008. p. 153–64.

10. Yang F, Wu Z, Xu C. The feasibility and acceptability of promoting condom use among the families with HIV infected individuals. Chinese Journal of Epidemiology. 2001;22(5): 330–3.

11. Zheng X, Mei Z, Wang C. Residual risk research of HIV infection after blood screening in one county in China. Chinese Journal of Epidemiology. 2000 Feb;21(1):13.

12. AIDS, syphilis, hepatitis: Shanxi exposes case involving 2 tons of infected blood. Southern

Metropolis Daily. Guangzhou; 2000 Mar 31.

13. Wang L. AIDS in Henan [Translated and quoted in Bandurski and Hala, 2010]. Dahe Daily. 2000 May 11.

14. People's Republic of China. Law of the People's Republic of China on Blood Donation. Dec 29, 1997.

15. Zhuang P. Fears over closure of blood plasma collection centres. South China Morning Post. Hong Kong; 2011 Aug 9.

16. Rogowska-Szadkowska D. Consequences of the commercialisation of plasma and blood in China. Przegl Epidemiol. 2011;65:515–9.

17. Gao X, Cui Q, Shi X, Su J, Peng Z, Chen X, et al. Prevalence and trend of hepatitis C virus infection among blood donors in Chinese mainland: a systematic review and meta-analysis. BMC Infectious Diseases. 2011;11(1):1.

18. Shan J. Better testing to secure safe blood supply. China Daily. Beijing; 2015 Jan 12.

19. Erwin K. The Circulatory System: Blood Procurement, AIDS, and the Social Body in China. Medical Anthropology Quarterly. 2006;20(2):139–59.

20. Rosenthal E. I Had to Help Them. Good Housekeeping. 2012 Jul 30.

21. Xiao Y, Kristensen S, Sun J, Lu L, Vermund SH. Expansion of HIV/AIDS in China: Lessons from Yunnan Province. Social Science & Medicine. 2007 Feb;64(3):665–75.

22. Monitoring the AIDS Pandemic. AIDS in Asia: Face the Facts. 2004.

23. Nelson KE, Celentano DD, Eiumtrakol S, Hoover DR, Beyrer C, Suprasert S, et al. Changes in sexual behavior and a decline in HIV infection among young men in Thailand [see comments]. N Engl J Med. 1996;335(5):297–303.

24. Rou K, Wu Z, Sullivan SG, Li F, Guan J, Xu C, et al. A five-city trial of a behavioural intervention to reduce sexually transmitted disease/HIV risk among sex workers in China. AIDS. 2007;21:S95–101.

25. Jeffreys E, Su G. China's 100 Per Cent Condom Use Program: Customising the Thai Experience. Asian Studies Review. 2011 Sep;35(3):315–33.

26. World Health Organization, Regional Office for the Western Pacific. Experiences of 100% condom use programme in selected countries of Asia. Manila: World Health Organization, Regional Office for the Western Pacific; 2004.

27. State Council of the Republic of China. Chinese National Medium-and Long-Term Strategic Plan for HIV/AIDS Prevention and Control (1998–2010). Beijing; 1998 Oct.

28. Jie S, Yu DB. Governmental policies on HIV infection in China. Cell Research. 2005;15(11):903–7.

29. Bezlova A. AIDS No Longer Taboo, But Still Sensitive Topic. Inter Press Service. Beijing; 2001 Nov 16.

30. Feckler M. UNsAnnan: China Has No Time to Lose in Curbing Spread of AIDS. Associated Press, via CDC, via TheBody.com. Zhejiang; 2002 Oct 14.

31. Clinton B. Frontline: The Age of AIDS. 2005.

32. Xinhua. China Reports New HIV/AIDS Statistics. Xinhua. Beijing; 2001 Aug 23.

33. UNAIDS. HIV/AIDS: China's Titanic Peril, 2002. Update of the AIDS Situation and Needs Assessment Report. Beijing: June; 2002.

34. Rosenthal E. U.N. Publicly Chastises China for Inaction on H.I.V. Epidemic. The New York Times. 2002 Jun 28.

35. Page J. U.N. Says China Faces AIDS Catastrophe. Reuters. Beijing; 2002 Jun 29.

36. Human Rights Watch. Locked doors: the human rights of people living with HIV/AIDS in China. Human Rights Watch; 2003 Sep. Report No.: Vol 15, 7C.

37. Wu Y. Seizing the Opportunity to Search Further, Accelerating the Work of HIV/AIDS Prevention and control in an All-around Way. National Conference of HIV/AIDS Prevention and control; 2004 Apr 4; Beijing.

38. Sun J, Liu H, Li H, Wang L, Guo H, Shan D, et al. Contributions of international cooperation projects to the HIV/AIDS response in China. International Journal of Epidemiology. 2010 Dec 1;39(Supplement 2):ii14–20.

39. Ma W, Detels R, Feng Y, Wu Z, Shen L, Li Y, et al. Acceptance of and barriers to voluntary HIV counselling and testing among adults in Guizhou province, China. AIDS (London, England). 2007;21(Suppl 8):S129.

40. Wu Z, Rou K, Xu C, Lou W, Detels R. Acceptability of HIV/AIDS counseling and testing among premarital couples in China. AIDS Education & Prevention. 2005;17(1):12–21.

41. Ministry of Health AIDS Expert Advisory Committee, Epidemiology and Intervention Management Group. Report on HIV Screening among Key Populations in Henan Province. Beijing: Ministry of Health, PRC; 2005 Sep.

42. AFP. Chinese jailed over AIDS secret. Sydney Morning Herald. Beijing; 2003 Oct 6.

43. Morgan D, Mahe C, Mayanja B, Okongo JM, Lubega R, Whitworth JA. HIV-1 infection in rural Africa: is there a difference in median time to AIDS and survival compared with that in industrialized countries? AIDS. 2002;16(4):597–603.

44. UNAIDS, World Health Organization. UNAIDS/WHO policy statement on HIV testing. UNAIDS; 2004.

45. UNAIDS. Fact Sheet: Revised HIV Estimates. UNAIDS; 2007.

46. Zhang D, Meng S, Xu P, Lu H, Zhuang M, Wu G, et al. Experience of Offering HIV Rapid Testing to At-Risk Patients in Community Health Centers in Eight Chinese Cities. PLoS ONE. 2014 Jan 28;9(1):e86609.

47. Moon S, Leemput LV, Durier N, Jambert E, Dahmane A, Jie Y, et al. Out-of-pocket costs of AIDS care in China: are free antiretroviral drugs enough? AIDS Care. 2008 Sep 1;20(8):984–94.

48. Wu Z, Zhao Y, Ge X, Mao Y, Tang Z, Shi CX, et al. Simplified HIV Testing and Treatment in China: Analysis of Mortality Rates Before and After a Structural Intervention. PLoS Med. 2015 Sep 8;12(9):e1001874.

49. Tang H, Mao Y, Shi CX, Han J, Wang L, Xu J, et al. Baseline CD4 Cell Counts of Newly Diagnosed HIV Cases in China: 2006–2012. PLoS ONE. 2014 Jun 5;9(6):e96098.

50. Wu Z, Zhao Y, Ge X, Mao Y, Tang Z, Shi CX, et al. Simplified HIV Testing and Treatment in China: Analysis of Mortality Rates Before and After a Structural Intervention. PLoS Med. 2015 Sep;12(9):e1001874.

51. Pang L, Hao Y, Mi G, Wang C, Luo W, Rou K, et al. Effectiveness of first eight methadone maintenance treatment clinics in China. AIDS. 2007;21:S103–7.

52. Zhang F, Dou Z, Ma Y, Zhang Y, Zhao Y, Zhao D, et al. Effect of earlier initiation of antiretroviral treatment and increased treatment coverage on HIV-related mortality in China: a national observational cohort study. The Lancet Infectious Diseases. 2011 Jul;11(7):516–24.

53. Ministry of Health, People's Republic of China, UNAIDS. 2005 Update on the HIV/AIDS Epidemic and Response in China. Beijing: National Center for AIDS/STD Prevention and Control, China CDC; 2006 Jan.

54. Poon AN, Li Z, Wang N, Hong Y. Review of HIV and other sexually transmitted infections among female sex workers in China. AIDS Care. 2011 Jun;23(sup1):5–25.

55. Chow EPF, Muessig KE, Yuan L, Wang Y, Zhang X, Zhao R, et al. Risk Behaviours among Female Sex Workers in China: A Systematic Review and Data Synthesis. Operario D, editor. PLoS ONE. 2015 Mar 27;10(3):e0120595.

56. Pisani E. The Wisdom of Whores: Bureaucrats, Brothels and the Business of AIDS. Granta Books; 2008. 288 p.

57. Chow JC. China's Billion Dollar Aid Appetite. Foreign Policy. 2010;19.

58. Huang Y, Ping J. The Global Funds China Legacy. Washington DC: Council on Foreign Relations.

59. Ban K. The stigma factor. Washington Times. Washington DC; 2008 Aug 6.

60. Wang Q, Suo L, Li X, Zhang B. History and current cultural background of men who have sex

with men in China. J of Pub Health and Prev Med. 2006;17(5):44–5.

61. UNAIDS. The China Stigma Index Report, 2009. Beijing: Joint United Nations Programme on HIV/AIDS; 2009.

62. Kaiser Family Foundation. 2009 Survey of Americans on HIV/AIDS: Summary of Findings on the Domestic Epidemic. Washington DC: Kaiser Family Foundation; 2009 Apr.

63. Human Rights Watch. China: Locked Doors : the Human Rights of People Living with HIV/AIDS in China. Human Rights Watch; 2003 Sep. Report No.: 15/7C.

64. National Center for AIDS/STD Control and Prevention. Survey report on discrimination against people living with HIV/AIDS. Beijing: China CDC; 2014 Oct.

65. Lau M. This is the last place to hide: 24 year-old Chinese man with HIV moves 4,700km from home to avoid the stigma of revealing his illness. South China Morning Post. Hong Kong; 2015 Dec 8.

66. An AIDS orphan's one-person primary school. Peninsula Morning Post. 2011 Nov 9.

67. Jiemian.com. Villagers vote to expel a HIV-positive child, stigma is still prevalent in China. Current politis in China, Interface news. [Internet]. Jiemian.com. 2014. Available from: http://www.jiemian.com/article/216781.html

68. National Center for AIDS/STD Control and Prevention, International Labor Organization. HIV and AIDS related employment discrimination in China. NCAIDS; 2011 Jan.

69. Cheng Y. AIDS Employment Discrimination Case First in China to Receive Compensation. Asia Catalyst. 2013.

70. Li Y, Zhang M. HIV carrier sues hospital for refusing surgery. China Daily. Tianjin; 2013 Mar 5.

71. Wu Z, Detels R, Ji G, Xu C, Rou K, Ding H, et al. Diffusion of HIV/AIDS knowledge, positive attitudes, and behaviors through training of health professionals in China. AIDS Educ Prev. 2002 Oct;14(5):379–90.

72. Liu ZF, Mei ZQ, Zheng XW, others. Investigation of HIV infection among plasma donors in three illegal plasma collection places in central China. Zhonghua Liu Xing Bing Xue Za Zhi. 2000;21(466):7.

73. Li L, Sun G, Liang S, Li J, Li T, Wang Z, et al. Different Distribution of HIV-1 Subtype and Drug Resistance Were Found among Treatment Naïve Individuals in Henan, Guangxi, and Yunnan Province of China. PLoS ONE. 2013 Oct 3;8(10):e75777.

74. Zhang L, Chow EP, Jing J, Zhuang X, Li X, He M, et al. HIV prevalence in China: integration of surveillance data and a systematic review. The Lancet Infectious Diseases. 2013;13(11):955–63.

75. Bai X, Xu J, Yang J, Yang B, Yu M, Gao Y, et al. HIV prevalence and high-risk sexual behaviours among MSM repeat and first-time testers in China: implications for HIV prevention. Journal of the International AIDS Society. 2014 Jul 2;17(1).

76. China National Center for AIDS/STD Control and Prevention. Baseline survey of MSM cohorts in five cities. Internal report. Division of Epidemiology, National Center for AIDS/STD Control and Prevention.; 2013.

图书在版编目（CIP）数据

中国公共卫生：艾滋病防治实践 =HIV/AIDS in China: Beyond the Numbers：英文 / 吴尊友主编. —北京：人民卫生出版社，2016
ISBN 978-7-117-22864-0

Ⅰ. ①中… Ⅱ. ①吴… Ⅲ. ①获得性免疫缺陷综合征－防治－中国－英文 Ⅳ. ①R512.91

中国版本图书馆 CIP 数据核字（2016）第 144206 号

| 人卫智网 | www.ipmph.com | 医学教育、学术、考试、健康，购书智慧智能综合服务平台 |
| 人卫官网 | www.pmph.com | 人卫官方资讯发布平台 |

中国公共卫生：艾滋病防治实践（英文）

主　　编：吴尊友
出版发行：人民卫生出版社（中继线 010-59780011）
地　　址：北京市朝阳区潘家园南里 19 号
邮　　编：100021
E - mail：pmph @ pmph.com
购书热线：010-59787592　010-59787584　010-65264830
印　　刷：北京盛通印刷股份有限公司
经　　销：新华书店
开　　本：710×1000　1/16　印张：12
字　　数：209 千字
版　　次：2016 年 6 月第 1 版　2017 年 1 月第 1 版第 2 次印刷
标准书号：ISBN 978-7-117-22864-0/R·22865
打击盗版举报电话：010-59787491　E-mail：WQ @ pmph.com
（凡属印装质量问题请与本社市场营销中心联系退换）

52检